Biology of Personality Disorders

EDITED BY
Kenneth R. Silk, M.D.

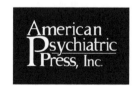

American Psychiatric Press, Inc.

WASHINGTON, DC
LONDON, ENGLAND

mi d tou

Copyright © 1998 American Psychiatric Press, Inc.
First Edition   01   00   99   4
ALL RIGHTS RESERVED
Manufactured in the United States of America on acid-free paper

American Psychiatric Press, Inc.
1400 K Street, N.W.
Washington, DC   20005
www.appi.org

Library of Congress Cataloging-in-Publication Data

Biology of personality disorders / edited by Kenneth R. Silk.
        p.   cm. — (Review of psychiatry series)
    Includes bibliographical references and index.
    ISBN 0-88048-835-2
    1. Personality disorders—Physiological aspects.   2. Personality
disorders—Treatment.   3. Neuroses—Physiological aspects.
    I. Silk, Kenneth R., 1944–   II. Series.
    [DNLM: 1. Personality Disorders.   WM 190 B6156 1998]
    616.85′8—dc21
    DNLM/DLC
    for Library of Congress   98-10615
                                                                                       CIP

British Library Cataloguing in Publication Data
A CIP record is available from the British Library.

4/6/2000

Biology of Personality Disorders

Review of Psychiatry Series

John M. Oldham, M.D., and
Michelle B. Riba, M.D., Series Editors

Contents

Contributors

C. Robert Cloninger, M.D. Wallace Renard Professor of Psychiatry and Genetics, Washington University School of Medicine, St. Louis, Missouri

Emil F. Coccaro, M.D. Professor and Director, Clinical Neuroscience Research Unit, Department of Psychiatry, MCP-Hahnemann School of Medicine, Allegheny University of the Health Sciences, Philadelphia, Pennsylvania

Robert Grossman, M.D. Assistant Professor, Department of Psychiatry, Mount Sinai School of Medicine, New York, New York

Ronald Heslegrave, Ph.D. Associate Professor of Psychiatry, Department of Psychiatry, Director of Research, St. Michael's/Wellesley Central Hospitals' Mental Health Service, University of Toronto, Toronto, Ontario

Richelle Kirrane, M.D. Fellow, Department of Psychiatry, Mount Sinai School of Medicine, New York, New York

Harold Koenigsberg, M.D. Associate Professor, New York Hospital–Cornell Medical Center, Department of Psychiatry, Westchester Division, White Plains, New York

Paul S. Links, M.D. Arthur Sommer Rotenberg Chair in Suicide Studies, Professor of Psychiatry, Department of Psychiatry, St. Michael's/Wellesley Central Hospitals' Mental Health Service, University of Toronto, Toronto, Ontario

Antonia S. New, M.D. Assistant Professor, Department of Psychiatry, Mount Sinai School of Medicine, New York, New York

Sherie Novotny, M.D. Fellow, Department of Psychiatry, Mount Sinai School of Medicine, New York, New York

John M. Oldham, M.D. Director, New York State Psychiatric Institute; Professor and Vice Chairman, Department of Psychiatry, Columbia University College of Physicians and Surgeons, New York, New York

Joel Paris, M.D. Professor and Chair, Department of Psychiatry, McGill University; Institute for Community and Family Psychiatry, Montréal, Québec

Michelle B. Riba, M.D. Clinical Associate Professor of Psychiatry and Associate Chair for Education and Academic Affairs, Department of Psychiatry, University of Michigan Health System, Ann Arbor, Michigan

Larry J. Siever, M.D. Professor, Department of Psychiatry, Mount Sinai School of Medicine, New York, New York

Kenneth R. Silk, M.D. Associate Professor of Psychiatry and Associate Chair for Clinical and Administrative Affairs, Department of Psychiatry, University of Michigan Medical Center, Ann Arbor, Michigan

John Villella, M.Sc. Undergraduate Summer Scholarship Student, Medical Student, University of Toronto, St. Michael's/ Wellesley Central Hospitals' Mental Health Service, Toronto, Ontario

Introduction to the Review of Psychiatry Series

John M. Oldham, M.D., and Michelle B. Riba, M.D.,
Series Editors

Beginning with 1998, the annual Review of Psychiatry adopts a new format. What were individual sections bound together in a large volume will be published only as independent monographs. Each monograph provides an update on a particular topic. Readers may then selectively purchase those monographs of particular interest to them. Last year, Volume 16 was available in the large volume and individual monographs, and the individually published sections were immensely successful. We think this new format adds flexibility and convenience to the always popular series.

Our goal is to maintain the overall mission of this series—that is, to provide useful and current clinical information, linked to new research evidence. For 1998 we have selected topics that overlap and relate to each other: 1) Psychopathology and Violent Crime, 2) New Treatments for Chemical Addictions, 3) Psychological Trauma, 4) Biology of Personality Disorders, 5) Child Psychopharmacology, and 6) Interpersonal Psychotherapy. All of the editors and chapter authors are experts in their fields. The monographs capture the current state of knowledge and practice while providing guideposts to future lines of investigation.

We are indebted to Helen ("Sam") McGowan for her dedication and skill and to Linda Gacioch for all of her help. We are indebted to the American Psychiatric Press, Inc., under the leadership of Carol C. Nadelson, M.D., who has supported this important and valued review series. We thank Claire Reinburg, Pamela Harley, Ron McMillen, and the APPI staff for all their generous assistance.

Foreword

Kenneth R. Silk, M.D.

Fifteen years ago, the idea of a major text in the Review of Psychiatry devoted to the biology of personality disorders would have been unthinkable. Although the concept of a separate axis for the personality disorders was put forward in 1980 in DSM-III (American Psychiatric Association 1980), the reasons for placing the personality disorders on a separate axis remain unclear. It has been suggested that DSM-III and its successive editions were designed to be primarily atheoretical. Nonetheless, there was the notion that the Axis I disorders would eventually be found to have significant etiological roots in biological predispositions and mechanisms (i.e., nature), whereas the personality disorders continued to be viewed as the result of primarily external events and the interpersonal behaviors and reactions around and to these events (i.e., environment and nurture). In 1983 this idea was reflected in a paper (Auchincloss and Michels 1983) that suggested that psychoanalysis's main area of expertise might be in the treatment of personality disorders. Although the authors did not imply that other disorders should not be treated with psychoanalysis, they nonetheless seem to have been reflecting the then-prevalent idea that while there certainly were alternative or adjunctive treatments to psychotherapy when it came to most Axis I disorders, the major mode of intervention for Axis II disorders was still psychotherapy and psychoanalytic psychotherapy. These assumptions with respect to differences between axes in the role of biology in etiology and treatment persisted despite evidence and argument to the contrary (Gunderson and Pollack 1985).

Ten years ago a number of different biological studies and theories with respect to the personality disorders began to emerge. These biological studies and theories grew out of a series of empirical examinations that tried to compare or contrast specific personality disorders with what were thought to be their near-neighbor Axis I disorders (Silk 1994a). For example, the argument was made that personality disorders, especially borderline personality disorder (BPD), are atypical manifestations of Axis I disorders such as cyclothymic disorder or bipolar II disorder (Akiskal et al. 1985a), although similar arguments might also be made with respect to schizotypal personality disorder (SPD) and schizophrenia; avoidant personality disorder and social phobia; histrionic personality disorder and somatization disorder; and paranoid personality disorder and delusional disorder or schizophrenia, paranoid type. This issue is raised not to try to argue it one way or the other but simply to direct attention to how the relationship between Axis I and Axis II was viewed at that time and how that thinking drove the first generation of biological studies of personality disorders.

These initial, first-generation biological studies sought to understand how biological processes in specific personality disorders were similar or dissimilar to biological processes in what were thought to be their near-neighbor Axis I disorders. Thus many of the early biological studies into BPD sought to appreciate better whether biological indices such as the dexamethasone suppression test (DST) or time of onset of rapid eye movement (REM) sleep distinguished these patients from patients with mood disorders, primarily major depressive disorder (Akiskal et al. 1985b; Baxter et al. 1984; Benson et al. 1990; Carroll et al. 1981; McNamara et al. 1984; Reynolds et al. 1985). The results of these studies, though interesting, did not lead to clear conclusions with respect to either whether the personality disorder was some atypical form of an Axis I disorder or what might be the underlying disturbed biological mechanisms in a specific personality disorder (Silk 1994a).

Biological researchers and theoreticians then turned their attention in a slightly different direction. Researchers turned to what have been called second-generation biological studies, studies that seek to better appreciate what might be the biological underpinnings of dimensions of psychopathology frequently found to be disrupted in patients across the personality disorders rather than attempting to study biological abnormalities in a single personality disorder. Led by the theoretical proposals of Cloninger (Cloninger 1987; Cloninger et al. 1993) and Siever and Davis (1991), researchers set out to look at possible biological disturbances in cognition, impulsivity and aggression, affective lability, and chronic anxiety among patients with personality disorders. This text attempts to provide an overview of the work undertaken to explore the biology of the dimensions that make up personality and in turn personality disorders.

In the first chapter, Coccaro reviews the existing data with regard to neurotransmitter correlates of personality in both healthy individuals and those with personality disorders. Unlike other reviews of this general topic area, this chapter is organized by type of neurotransmitter rather than by diagnosis or behavioral indexes. Although most of the research to date supports the inverse relationship between serotonin and impulsive aggression, a body of data that may implicate other neurotransmitters such as dopamine and norepinephrine in aggressive and impulsive behavior is also beginning to accumulate. Acetylcholine may play a key role in some aspects of emotional lability, and dopamine certainly is involved in abnormal, odd, or unusual cognitions or schizotypy. Many of these neurotransmitter studies are quite elegant, reflecting the application of the most recent biological techniques to the study of neurotransmitters and personality. And yet, as in most areas of psychiatry, much more needs to be known, even while we may marvel at the amount of information discovered within the last 5–10 years.

In Chapter 2, Siever and colleagues reveal, as they review the literature, the degree of sophistication in research strategies into the biology of the personality disorders. This chapter serves as an accompaniment to Coccaro's chapter in that Siever and colleagues look at research strategies that explore biological areas other than the neurotransmitters. Both older and newer strategies that carefully examine the hypothalamic-pituitary-adrenal (HPA) axis are reviewed, with attention paid to the effects of early and profound trauma on HPA functioning and feedback. Neuroimaging strategies that include computed tomography (CT) and magnetic resonance imaging (MRI) allow observation of brain structures with improving spatial resolution and sharper definition between gray and white matter. Positron-emission tomography (PET), single photon emission computed tomography (SPECT), and functional magnetic resonance imaging (fMRI) permit visualization of regional patterns of brain activation, and magnetic resonance spectroscopy (MRS) can localize specific neurochemical processes within the functioning brain. Siever et al. review the variety and sophistication of both past and current techniques and point to future strategies that should assist us in solving some of the anatomic and neurofunctional mysteries surrounding personality pathology. Cognitive science strategies include the study of cognitive processes such as executive function, learning, abstraction, language, and attention. New tools of cognitive neuroscience permit researchers to investigate critically cognitive processes in patients with personality disorders and link these processes to specific personality traits. Thus a new approach to study the biological basis of these disorders is to investigate the neurochemistry and pharmacology of cognition and cognitive impairment. Siever et al. review the current data with respect to both SPD and BPD. Finally, this chapter considers the arena of candidate gene strategies and presents some important and exciting findings with respect to impulsive aggression, serotonin, and genetic polymorphism.

In Chapter 3, Cloninger reviews the studies conducted to date that support his seven-factor model of personality, a model that includes factors of both temperament (i.e., nature) and character (i.e., nurture). First, Cloninger describes a model of the genetic structure of personality (temperament and character) based on twin and adoption studies of personality in humans. Then, based on neuropharmacological studies of humans and animals, he proposes a psychobiological model of learning abilities that underlie human personality traits. Finally, he reviews his own work and that of many independent investigators who have evaluated the psychometric properties of quantitative tests for measuring personality and its disorders in the general population and many clinical samples (Cloninger 1994). More recently, extensive work has been carried out by many investigators to characterize the neuroanatomy, neuropsychology, neurochemistry, and neurogenetics of human personality using the two tests developed by Cloninger and colleagues, the Tridimensional Personality Questionnaire (TPQ) (Cloninger et al. 1987; Stallings et al. 1996) and the more comprehensive Temperament and Character Inventory (TCI) (Cloninger et al. 1994) to support a neurobiological basis for the four dimensions of temperament: harm avoidance, novelty seeking, reward dependence, and persistence (Cloninger et al. 1993).

In the final two chapters we move away from basic science principles and toward utilizing some of these principles in the treatment of patients with personality disorders. Links and colleagues present a novel approach to the pharmacological treatment of patients with personality disorders. Much of the pharmacological treatment of these patients remains empirical and can be seen as conducted on a trial and error basis. Links et al. review what we know about specific pharmacological treatments for these disorders and discuss current ways to approach and consider pharmacological agents for individuals with personality disorders. Then, in a novel and interesting way, the authors suggest an outcome-focused model for pharmacological treatment. The outcome-focused model is based on specific measurable behavioral targets such as self-harm behavior, repeated suicidal behavior, and treatment adherence, as well as quality of life and functional outcome measures that, considered together, might drive the choice of a particular pharmacological agent. The choices should also be informed by the relationship of the specific Axis II disorder to an Axis I disorder and should follow logical principles with respect to what we know about the biology of personality disorders. Links and colleagues propose this model for the current treatment of patients with personality disorders but also suggest that the tenets of this model be applied to evaluate the utility of a given pharmacological agent in pharmacological treatment studies.

Finally, Paris attempts to put it all together in considering the significance of biological research for a biopsychosocial model of the personality disorders. The biopsychosocial model (Engel 1980) assumes that constitution, experience, and the social environment are all crucial in the etiology of mental disorders, though as our knowledge expands we may assume that biology plays the largest role. Genetic predispositions determine which kinds of disorders individuals may develop, whereas psychosocial factors function as precipitants of pathology. This approach, which corresponds to the diathesis-stress model of mental disorders (Monroe and Simons 1991), suggests that genes shape predispositions, whereas environmental stressors determine whether underlying vulnerabilities develop into overt disorders. The diathesis-stress model is particularly applicable to the personality disorders. The diatheses for these conditions are trait profiles. Traits determine what kinds of disorders will probably develop, and when these traits are unusually intense, they may be risk factors for pathology (Siever and Davis 1991). The stressors that can elicit personality disorders range widely from psychological adversities to social disintegration (Paris 1996). In detailing each one of these contributions, traits, and temperaments as a result of genetic predisposition and social, cultural, and adaptational factors, as well systemic (environmental, familial, and interpersonal) responses to stress, Paris goes on to show how this model has implications not only for the treatment of personality disorders but also for the methodological structure of research into the personality disorders.

This text then travels from the molecular level of the gene through structural brain chemistry and cognitive neuroscience, to neurotransmitters, to adaptational ability, and finally to the effects of life's experiences to propose that the biological underpinnings, while new and exciting to the researcher, can also inform the types of pharmacological agents and psychotherapeutic interventions that clinicians may employ. In the last 15–20 years we have traveled an extraordinarily long distance in our appreciation of the role of biology in the origins of the personality disorders, and we have made great strides in our understanding of some of those biological mechanisms. But ultimately we have really only begun to isolate and consider certain likely suspects in their relation to the biology of personality disorders. The identification of the suspects combined with the advances in sophisticated neurobiological and molecular probes should lead us toward a much greater understanding of the biological basis of personality. These discoveries should then help us to develop and refine more specific and effective treatments for a large group of patients whose current treatment remains fraught with frustrating limitations (Silk 1994b).

References

Akiskal HS, Chen SE, David GC, et al: Borderline: an adjective in search of a noun. J Clin Psychiatry 46:41–48, 1985a

Akiskal HS, Yerevanian BI, Davis GC: The nosologic status of borderline personality: clinical and polysomnographic study. Am J Psychiatry 142:192–198, 1985b

American Psychiatric Association: Diagnostic and Statistical Manual of Mental Disorders, 3rd Edition. Washington, DC, American Psychiatric Association, 1980

Auchincloss EL, Michels RM: Psychoanalytic theory of character, in Current Perspectives in Personality Disorders. Edited by Frosch J. Washington, DC, American Psychiatric Press, 1983, pp 2–17

Baxter L, Edell W, Gerner R, et al: Dexamethasone suppression test and Axis I diagnoses of inpatients with DSM-III borderline personality disorder. J Clin Psychiatry 45:150–153, 1984

Benson KL, King R, Gordon D, et al: Sleep patterns in borderline personality disorder. J Affective Disord 18:267–273, 1990

Carroll BJ, Greden JF, Feinberg M, et al: Neuroendocrine evaluation of depression in borderline patients. Psychiatr Clin North Am 4:89–99, 1981

Cloninger CR: A systematic method for clinical description and classification of personality variants. Arch Gen Psychiatry 44:579–588, 1987

Cloninger CR: Temperament and personality. Curr Opin Neurobiol 4:226–277, 1994

Cloninger CR, Svrakic DM, Pryzbeck TR: A psychobiological model of temperament and character. Arch Gen Psychiatry 50:975–990, 1993

Cloninger CR, Przybeck TR, Svrakic DM, et al: The Temperament and Character Inventory (TCI): A Guide to Its Development and Use. St. Louis, MO, Washington University Center for Psychobiology of Personality, 1994

Engel GL: The clinical application of the biopsychosocial model. Am J Psychiatry 137:535–544, 1980

Gunderson JG, Pollack WS: Conceptual risks of Axis I–II division, in Biologic Response Styles: Clinical Implications. Edited by Klar H,

Siever LJ. Washington, DC, American Psychiatric Press, 1985, pp 81–95

McNamara E, Reynolds CS III, Soloff PH, et al: EEG sleep evaluation of depression in borderline patients. Am J Psychiatry 141:182–186, 1984

Monroe SM, Simons AD: Diathesis-stress theories in the context of life stress research. Psychol Bull 110:406–425, 1991

Paris J: Social Factors in the Personality Disorders. New York, Cambridge University Press, 1996

Reynolds CF, Soloff PH, Kupfer DJ, et al: Depression in borderline patients: a prospective EEG sleep study. Psychiatry Res 14:1–15, 1985

Siever LJ, Davis KL: Psychobiological perspective on the personality disorders. Am J Psychiatry 148:1647–1658, 1991

Silk KR: From first- to second-generation biological studies of borderline personality disorder, in Biological and Neurobehavioral Studies of Borderline Personality Disorder. Edited by Silk K. Washington, DC, American Psychiatric Press, 1994a, pp xvii–xxix

Silk KR: Implications of biological research for clinical work with borderline patients, in Biological and Neurobehavioral Studies of Borderline Personality Disorder. Edited by Silk K. Washington, DC, American Psychiatric Press, 1994b, pp 227–240

Stallings MC, Hewitt JK, Cloninger CR, et al: Genetic and environmental structure of the Tridimensional Personality Questionnaire: three or four temperament dimensions? J Pers Soc Psychol 70:127–140, 1996

Chapter 1

Neurotransmitter Function in Personality Disorders

Emil F. Coccaro, M.D.

The notion that disorders of personality are due purely to developmental or other environmental factors has been refuted over the past 15–20 years by accumulating data from psychobiological research studies. First, various dimensions of personality have been shown to be moderately heritable in twin studies (Plomin et al. 1994). Accordingly, then, to a substantial degree, individual differences in personality must be influenced by genetic, and therefore biological, factors, and these ideas are expanded upon further in Chapters 2 and 3 of this text. Second, various dimensions of personality have been shown to correlate with various measures of biological function (Coccaro and Siever 1995). In general, these correlations between personality "styles" and biological measures have been reported primarily with indexes of specific neurotransmitter function.

In this chapter, we review the existing data, specifically with regard to the neurotransmitter correlates of personality in both healthy individuals and people with personality disorders. This chapter can serve as an accompaniment to Chapter 2 by Siever and colleagues, which focuses on nonneurotransmitter biological correlates of personality disorders. Unlike other reviews in this general topic area, this review is organized by type of neurotransmitter rather than by diagnosis or behavioral indexes. Although such an organization for the chapter might tend to result in a fairly technical review of the literature, we make every effort to summarize pertinent points and refer back to clinical phenomena where applicable, though much of this research remains to be transcribed to the clinical arena. Rarely, however, has this topic been approached in this particular manner, and we hope that this chapter might become a resource for the researcher, as well as the clinician who seeks to better appreciate what we understand about the roles of neurotransmitters in normal and abnormal personality functioning.

Serotonin

The most heavily researched neurotransmitter with regard to personality and personality disorder is serotonin (5-hydroxy-tryptamine [5-HT]). Over the course of the last 20 years, research in this area has suggested a strong role for 5-HT in aggression and impulsivity. These studies repeatedly reveal that 5-HT levels are *inversely* related to aggression and/or impulsivity. Thus, the lower the 5-HT, the greater the propensity to aggression or impulsivity. Although some studies suggest that 5-HT levels may be more closely (inversely) correlated with impulsivity than with aggression, most studies in fact report a relationship between 5-HT and both impulsivity *and* aggression (e.g., impulsive aggression) rather than with one personality dimension or the other. One of the most remarkable aspects of this literature is the general consistency of these findings across different study samples and using various assessments of 5-HT function.

Evidence for a role of 5-HT in aggression was first reported in studies of nonprimate mammals such as mice and rats (Valzelli 1980). In these studies, experimental reduction or enhancement of 5-HT was associated with an increase or decrease, respectively, in aggressive response in these lower mammals. In the following sections, we review the variety of human studies that generally confirm this inverse relationship between 5-HT and aggression.

Cerebrospinal Fluid Monoamine Metabolite Studies

The major 5-HT metabolite in the lumbar cerebrospinal fluid (CSF) is 5-hydroxyindoleacetic acid (5-HIAA), and 5-HIAA is measured in the CSF (CSF 5-HIAA). Because 5-HIAA is the metabolite of 5-HT, this index, CSF 5-HIAA, is thought to represent central turnover of 5-HT. This view is supported by the observation that CSF 5-HIAA is highly correlated with brain concentrations of 5-HIAA (Stanley et al. 1985). However, this interpretation of the relationship between CSF-HIAA and brain concentrations of 5-HT and 5-HIAA remains controversial. A more conservative interpretation suggests that CSF 5-HIAA represents an index of the number of viable 5-HT neurons in the central nervous system (CNS) (Murphy et al. 1990).

In the human, the first evidence of an inverse relationship between 5-HT and aggression was reported by Asberg et al. (1976) in their landmark study of CSF 5-HIAA in depressed patients as a function of history of suicide attempting behavior. In this study, a disproportionate number of depressed patients with histories of suicide attempts had categorically low CSF 5-HIAA concentrations. An even more impressive finding was that among suicide attempters, all who had made a suicide attempt classified as violent had categorically low CSF 5-HIAA concentrations. Two patients who ultimately killed themselves also had categorically low CSF 5-HIAA concentrations. Patients who had made nonviolent suicide attempts were approximately split between the classifications of categorically low and normal CSF 5-HIAA concentrations.

Three years later, Brown et al. (1979) reported a specific inverse relationship between CSF 5-HIAA concentrations and life history of actual aggressive behavior in 24 male subjects with personality disorders. The subjects were Navy recruits referred for fitness-for-duty evaluations. Personality disorder was assessed by DSM-II (American Psychiatric Association 1968), and subjects had a variety of personality diagnoses. The correlation between CSF 5-HIAA and life history of aggression was very strong ($r = -.78$, $P < .001$). In addition, CSF 5-HIAA was reduced among recruits with life histories of suicide attempts. In 1982 Brown et al. reported a replication study in 12 male Navy recruits with DSM-III (American Psychiatric Association 1980) borderline personality disorder. In this study CSF 5-HIAA and life history of aggression again were inversely correlated, but this inverse correlation was only at a trend level of significance for a two-tailed test ($r = -.53$, $N = 12$, $P < .08$). In addition, the psychopathic deviance (Pd) scale of the Minnesota Multiphasic Personality Inventory (MMPI) (Hathaway and McKinley 1943) was found to correlate inversely and significantly with CSF 5-HIAA ($r = -.77$, $P < .01$). In a subsequent analysis, Brown et al. (1982) demonstrated a trivariate relationship among aggression history, suicide history, and reduced CSF 5-HIAA levels. History of aggression and suicide attempt were correlated directly with each other, while each historical behavioral variable correlated inversely with CSF 5-HIAA levels.

The story of the inverse correlation between CSF 5-HIAA levels and impulsive behavior continued. In 1983 Linnoila et al. reported reduced CSF 5-HIAA levels in 28 impulsive, but not in 8 nonimpulsive, violent offenders (i.e., individuals who had committed murder or attempted murder or serious assault). Subjects who had committed impulsive acts of violence had not generally known the victim before the crime and had apparently not planned out the attack. All subjects had a history of alcoholism, but the subjects had been alcohol free for several months before the study. As in the Brown et al. (1979) study, personality disorders were assessed by DSM-II, and impulsive subjects had either antisocial or explosive personality diagnoses; nonimpulsive subjects had either paranoid or passive-aggressive personality diagnoses. The observation that impulsive, rather than nonimpulsive, aggression was associated with reduced CSF 5-HIAA concentration suggested that *impulsiveness* might be the more specific phenomenologic or behavioral correlate to 5-HT function. This hypothesis was explored further by Virkkunen et al. (1987) in a study of impulsive arsonists. Impulsive arsonists were fire setters who committed arson without an extensive plan and did so without concern for personal gain. Personality disorders in this study were assessed using DSM-III, and all of the impulsive arsonists also met criteria for borderline personality disorder. The arsonists had significantly reduced CSF 5-HIAA concentrations compared with normal volunteers. The CSF 5-HIAA concentrations of the arsonists were similar to those of the impulsive violent offenders. Since the common denominator for the reduced CSF 5-HIAA concentration finding appeared to be impulsivity as opposed to violence, these data suggested a primacy for impulsivity over aggression in relation to central 5-HT function. Evidence from later studies, described later in this chapter, however, suggests that the critical phenomenologic factor may be impulsive aggression rather than simply impulsivity alone.

The finding of reduced CSF 5-HIAA concentration in subjects with aggressive personality disorders generally has been replicated when the subjects studied were criminal offenders. However, when subjects with personality disorders without a history of criminal activity are studied, CSF 5-HIAA analyses are equivocal in terms of a relationship with aggression. For example, Gardner et al. (1990) reported no correlation between CSF 5-HIAA levels and life history of aggression in 17 female patients with borderline personality disorder. In a more recent study of 52 male and female subjects with personality disorders, half of whom were classified as self-mutilators, no correlation between CSF 5-HIAA concentration and measures of aggression or impulsivity was observed (Simeon et al. 1992). In addition, Coccaro and colleagues (1997a) reported no correlation between CSF 5-HIAA concentrations and life history measure of aggression in a study of 24 male and female subjects with personality disorders, and these researchers also reported no correlation between CSF 5-HIAA levels and self-reported tendency to assaultiveness in a different study of 22 male subjects with personality disorders (Coccaro et al., in press).

In contrast, a recent study of healthy volunteers reported a *positive* correlation between CSF 5-HIAA levels and self-reported outwardly directed aggression. The reason for the differential findings across populations is probably a function of the severity of aggressive behavior being measured. If 5-HT correlates inversely with aggression, it is likely that individuals with a history of the most severe aggression should have the lowest 5-HT function. Since CSF 5-HIAA is a relatively insensitive index of 5-HT activity, it is likely that only the most profound central 5-HT deficit would be reflected in lumber CSF 5-HIAA concentrations. Accordingly, in a cohort of less severely aggressive subjects, there will be fewer subjects with low CSF 5-HIAA levels, and then the ability to detect an inverse correlation will be difficult and the differences in CSF 5-HIAA concentrations among subjects smaller. Another possibility for the differential findings is that less severely aggressive subjects are better able to compensate for reductions in presynaptic 5-HT output by increasing the sensitivity of their postsynaptic 5-HT receptors. Under this model, the physiological responsivity to 5-HT stimulation is the critical factor in the 5-HT–to–aggression relationship, and thus there is no primary relationship between CSF 5-HIAA levels and measures of aggression. In this regard, it is noteworthy that in some samples in which CSF 5-HIAA concentrations did not correlate with measures of aggression, the studies also involved a pharmacological challenge, and in utilizing the challenge, an inverse correlation between a physiological response to 5-HT stimulation (e.g., prolactin response to fenfluramine) and measures of aggression was indeed found (Coccaro et al. 1997a, in press). Again, however, what is most important here is the general consistency of these findings—that is, the inverse relationship between CSF 5-HIAA levels and measures of impulsive aggression across different study samples and using various assessments of 5-HT function. This finding, among others, has led to research in the use of the selective serotonin reuptake inhibitors (SSRIs) to treat impulsivity among patients with and without personality disorders.

Pharmacological Challenge Studies

In pharmacological challenge studies, a physiological response (e.g., hormonal, behavioral, or thermal) to the acute administration of agents that activate central 5-HT synapses (or receptors) is assessed. Since these responses are dose related, the degree of response is interpreted as the physiological responsiveness of the central 5-HT synapses or receptors in relevant areas of the brain (Coccaro and Kavoussi 1994). In contrast to CSF 5-HIAA assessments, pharmacological challenge studies offer a dynamic view of central 5-HT activity and, at the same time, suggest a particular brain location (such as the hypothalamus for hormonal and thermal responses).

A variety of 5-HT pharmacological challenge studies have been performed in subjects with personality disorders in the context of the study of aggression. The first study in this area was reported by Coccaro et al. (1989). In this study, prolactin responses to the 5-HT releaser or uptake inhibitor *d,l*-fenfluramine (i.e., PRL[*d,l*-FEN]) were examined in 20 male subjects with personality disorder. Subjects with personality disorders were found to have reduced PRL(*d,l*-FEN) responses when compared with normal male volunteers, though not when compared with patients with mood disorders. Among the subtypes of personality disorder, only subjects with borderline personality disorder had reduced PRL(*d,l*-FEN) responses. This finding was actually more specific to a relationship with aggression. For example, among all subjects with personality disorders, those positive for the borderline diagnostic criteria of anger dyscontrol, self-damaging behavior, and impulsivity had significantly lower PRL(*d,l*-FEN) responses when compared with subjects who did not meet these specific diagnostic criteria. Not surprisingly, PRL(*d,l*-FEN) responses were inversely correlated with measures of aggression and impulsivity, specifically assaultiveness and irritability (which, in turn, correlated with impulsiveness). Again, when levels of assaultiveness and irritability were controlled for statistically, subjects with borderline personality disorder no longer appeared to have reduced PRL(*d,l*-FEN) responsiveness. This was true for other findings in this sample as well, such as the inverse relationship between PRL(*d,l*-FEN) responses and a past history of a suicide attempt and a past history of alcoholism. As with borderline personality disorder, each of these two factors correlated directly with the aggression and irritability variables. When levels of assaultiveness and irritability were controlled for statistically, subjects positive for either factor no longer appeared to have reduced PRL(*d,l*-FEN) responsiveness. Moreover, when each of these three factors was included in the same regression model, only the aggression and irritability variables contributed uniquely to the model. Accordingly, these data suggested that the strongest behavioral correlate of reduced PRL(d,l-FEN) responses, as an index of central 5-HT system function, was the type of irritable aggression that had shared variance with impulsivity (i.e., impulsive aggression).

An inverse relationship between the prolactin response to fenfluramine challenge and aggression has been replicated in several, though not all, studies of subjects with personality disorders. O'Keane et al. (1992) reported a reduction in PRL(d-FEN) responses in nine violent offenders with antisocial personality disorder when compared with nine healthy volunteers. Siever and Trestman (1993), extending the earlier report by Coccaro et al. (1989), reported a consistently strong inverse correlation between PRL(d,l-FEN) and self-reported assaultiveness (but not irritability) in a total of 32 subjects with personality disorders. Stein et al. (1996) reported reduced PRL(d,l-FEN) responses among nine subjects with compulsive personality disorders, but they also noted that this group effect was due to higher aggression scores among this cohort. New et al. (1997) reported reduced PRL(d,l-FEN) responses among subjects with personality disorders and a past history of suicidal or self-injurious behavior compared with subjects with personality disorders without this history. Further studies by Coccaro et al. (1996a, 1997a) that used d-fenfluramine confirmed an inverse correlation between PRL[d-FEN] responses and a life history of aggression (Coccaro et al. 1996a, 1997a) and laboratory measures of aggression (Coccaro et al. 1996a). In contrast, Fishbein et al. (1989) reported a positive relationship between PRL[d,l-FEN] responses and self-reported impulsiveness in 22 male patients with antisocial personality disorders and who abused drugs. Reasons for the differential relationship between PRL[d,l-FEN] and impulsiveness include the drug abusing nature of the population and the fact that the drug-free period was only a minimum of 5 days. A recent study by Bernstein and Handlesman (1995) suggests that selected drug abusing populations (e.g., cocaine abusers) demonstrate a positive, rather than an inverse, relationship between hormonal responses to 5-HT stimulation and measures of aggression. This finding is in contrast to results from subjects who abuse alcohol, where inverse relationships between hormonal responses to 5-HT stimulation (i.e., with metachlorophenylpiperazine [m-CPP]) and measures of aggression are reported (Handlesman et al. 1996; Moss et al. 1990). Again, however, we see here the almost universal finding of an inverse relationship between behavioral measures of impulsive aggression and a pharmacological challenge test that reveals low central 5-HT activity.

Pharmacological challenge studies of personality disorders using 5-HT agents other than fenfluramine are limited, but these few other studies generally support the hypothesis of an inverse relationship between 5-HT and measures of aggression. These studies used 5-HT agents including direct 5-HT agonists and 5-HT$_{1a}$ partial agonists. Moss et al. (1990) reported reduced prolactin responses to the postsynaptic 5-HT agonist PRL(m-CPP) in 15 male patients with antisocial personality disorder with comorbid alcohol abuse when compared with normal volunteers. An inverse correlation between PRL(m-CPP) responses and assaultiveness was also reported across all subjects. Although Coccaro et al. (in press) could not replicate this finding in 20 male and female subjects with personality disorders, the PRL(m-CPP) responses demonstrated had similar inverse correlations to those seen with PRL(d,l-FEN) responses in the subgroup of 10 male subjects in whom both PRL(m-CPP) and PRL(d,l-FEN) response data were available. This similarity was due to a strong intercorrelation between PRL(m-CPP) and PRL(d,l-FEN) responses in these subjects. In examining the 5-HT$_{1a}$ receptor, Coccaro et al. (1990) reported an inverse correlation between the prolactin response to the 5-HT$_{1a}$ partial agonist buspirone and self-reported assaultiveness and irritability in 10 subjects with personality disorders. A follow-up study using a more potent and selective 5-HT$_{1a}$ agonist, ipsapirone, also found an inverse correlation between measures of aggression and cortisol and thermal responses to ipsapirone in eight male subjects with personality disorders. PRL(d-FEN) responses were also found to correlate inversely with aggression in these same subjects.

Behavioral responses to 5-HT stimulation in subjects with personality disorders have not received as much attention as have the neuroendocrine responses. However, a recent study reported a significant reduction in anger in 12 subjects with borderline personality disorder after administration of m-CPP but not after administration of a placebo (Hollander et al. 1994). In addition, a reduction in fear was observed after the m-CPP administration in the male subjects with borderline personality disorder.

As our knowledge of which 5-HT receptor subtypes mediate physiological responses to 5-HT stimulation increases, we are better able to interpret the results of these studies. With regard to the fenfluramine challenge, the prolactin response to fenfluramine appears to be mediated, at the least, by 5-HT_{2a} and/or 5-HT_{2c} receptors. This finding is based on studies that demonstrate complete blockade of this prolactin response to pretreatment with 5-HT_{2a} or 5-HT_{2c} receptor antagonists such as ritanserin (Goodall et al. 1993) and amesergide (Coccaro et al. 1996b); however, there was no effective blockade of this response after pretreatment with the 5-HT_{1a} receptor antagonist pindolol (Park and Cowen 1995) or the 5-HT_3 receptor antagonist ondansetron (Coccaro et al. 1996c). These data do not rule out a role for other 5-HT receptor subtypes. However, there are no other 5-HT receptor antagonist probes available at this time for further study in humans. In contrast to fenfluramine, some evidence suggests that the prolactin response to m-CPP challenge is mediated by both 5-HT_{1a} and 5-HT_{2c} receptor activation. This belief is based on studies that demonstrate significant attenuation of the prolactin response to m-CPP after pretreatment with pindolol (Meltzer and Maes 1995) or ritanserin (Seibyl et al. 1991). Since m-CPP is itself an antagonist at the 5-HT_{2a} receptor site (Simansky and Schechter 1988), attenuation of prolactin responses by the 5-HT_{2a} or 5-HT_{2c} receptor antagonist ritanserin must be due to blockade at the 5-HT_{2c} site. Overall, these data suggest the possibility that inverse relationships between prolactin responses to fenfluramine and aggression (Coccaro et al. 1989, 1996a, 1997a; O'Keane et al. 1992; Siever and Trestman 1993) reflect signal transduction abnormalities at postsynaptic 5-HT_{2a} or 5-HT_{2c} receptor sites. The inverse relationships noted between prolactin responses to m-CPP and aggression (Handlesman et al. 1996; Moss et al. 1990) may reflect similar abnormalities at 5-HT_{1a} and 5-HT_{2c} receptor sites. Preliminary observations using partial 5-HT$_{1a}$ agonists (Coccaro et al. 1990, 1995) are consistent with a role for both pre- and postsynaptic 5-HT$_{1a}$ receptors (Coccaro et al. 1990, 1995) in aggressive behavior as manifested in subjects with personality disorders. Thus, as we move from the CSF to the molecular level, the inverse correlation between the 5-HT metabolite 5-HIAA, 5-HT activity, or 5-HT receptor activity and measures of impulsive aggression persists.

Platelet Serotonin Receptor and Blood Platelet Serotonin Studies

Receptor markers on circulating blood platelets have long been used as a model of 5-HT receptors in the CNS. Although these platelet 5-HT receptors are not innervated by 5-HT neurons, platelet 5-HT transporter sites and 5-HT$_{2a}$ receptor sites are essentially identical to the corresponding sites in the brain (Cook et al. 1994; Lesch et al. 1993).

Despite considerable platelet receptor work in other psychiatric populations, relatively little research in this area has been published on subjects with personality disorders. Simeon et al. (1992) reported an inverse correlation between the number of platelet ^{3}H-imipramine (5-HT transporter) binding sites and self-mutilation and impulsivity in 26 subjects with personality disorders and a history of self-mutilation; this inverse correlation was not found in subjects with personality disorders who were not self-mutilators. Recently, Coccaro and colleagues (1996d) reported that the number of platelet ^{3}H-paroxetine (5-HT transporter) binding sites was inversely correlated with life history of aggression in 24 male and female subjects with personality disorders. This finding suggests that the greater the life history of aggression, the fewer the number of presynaptic 5-HT transporter sites and the greater the chance of alteration in 5-HT function. These findings are consistent with what has been reported for 5-HT transporter binding in aggressive populations though not necessarily those with personality disorders (Bermaher et al. 1990; Marazziti et al. 1993; Stoff et al. 1987). Studies of the 5-HT$_{2a}$ receptor are also quite rare but less consistent in their results.

McBride et al. (1994) reported no differences between patients with major depression with and without comorbid borderline personality disorder among three measures of platelet 5-HT$_{2a}$ receptor activity. In another study by Coccaro and colleagues (1997b), the number and affinity of ^{125}I-LSD (5-HT$_{2a}$) binding sites in subjects with personality disorders was directly correlated with the self-reported tendency to be aggressive. The latter finding is consistent with what has been reported for 5-HT$_{2a}$ receptor binding in various subjects with histories of suicidal behavior (Biegon et al. 1990; Pandey et al. 1995).

Only one study involving blood or platelet 5-HT content is available in subjects with personality disorders (Mann et al. 1992). In this study, blood and platelet 5-HT content were examined in depressed subjects as a function of suicidal behavior. Among a subgroup of subjects, depressed patients with comorbid borderline personality disorder were reported to have higher whole blood 5-HT levels than controls. Among suicide attempters, depressed patients with comorbid borderline personality disorder had higher whole blood 5-HT concentrations than corresponding patients without comorbid borderline personality disorder. The meaning of this finding is unclear, however. First, the direction of the findings with blood platelet 5-HT is opposite to the direction of the findings reported with more centrally relevant measures of 5-HT function. Second, the latter finding (bipolar disorder versus nonbipolar disorder) did not hold up after controlling for the variability attributed to seasonality. Overall, these findings, as well as the relative case of obtaining samples for the assessment of 5-HT receptor binding sites and 5-HT content, suggest that more research in this area is warranted and needed, particularly among patients with personality disorders.

DNA Polymorphism Studies

Polymorphisms are different forms of DNA sequences that represent either anonymous DNA markers (for gene mapping purposes) or DNA markers of known genes that code for specific proteins. Work with specific polymorphic markers of candidate genes is now being applied to subjects with personality disorders, a topic that is also touched on in Chapter 2 of this text.

The first published study of polymorphisms that involved subjects with personality disorders examined the biallelic polymorphism for the tryptophan hydroxylase (TPH) gene in a population of Finnish violent offenders (Nielsen et al. 1994). Because TPH is the rate limiting step in the synthesis of 5-HT, TPH represents a logical candidate gene polymorphism to examine with respect to aggression in this highly violent population. Among impulsive violent offenders in this study, subjects with at least one copy of the L allele (i.e., LL or LU genotype) had significantly lower CSF 5-HIAA concentrations when compared with impulsive violent offenders with the UU genotype. This finding suggested an allelic correlation between the L allele and reduced CSF 5-HIAA levels in these subjects; the allelic correlation did not exist in nonviolent offenders or normal volunteers. However, since the TPH polymorphism is located in an intron (i.e., a noncoding DNA region), it is possible that this polymorphism might be in linkage disequilibrium with another, currently unknown, polymorphism, which accounts for the findings reported only in impulsive, as opposed to nonimpulsive, violent offenders. A second finding was that the presence of the L allele was associated with an increased frequency of a past history of suicide attempts across all violent offender subjects regardless of the presence of impulsivity. Given the strong evidence of reduced CSF 5-HIAA concentrations in suicidal individuals, this finding is difficult to reconcile with the first. Further study in this area with respect to both impulsivity and aggression is clearly warranted.

A second study of the TPH polymorphism in subjects with personality disorders was conducted by New et al. (in press). In this study, the tendency toward aggression as measured by self-report was examined as a function of TPH genotype in 40 white male subjects with personality disorders. Subjects with the LL genotype were found to have higher aggression scores than those with the LU or UU genotype. No relationship was noted between TPH genotype and history of suicide attempts; however, only 5 of the 40 subjects were positive for a history of suicide attempts. Although PRL(d,l-FEN) responses did not differ significantly as a function of genotype in the subgroup with this suicide attempt history, PRL(*d,l*-FEN) responses among those with the LL genotype were 30% lower than of those with the LU and UU genotypes. These data are promising and need to be replicated and extended in larger samples and with other 5-HT–related polymorphisms.

Thus we see that at all levels, even at the level of the genome, there is a correlation, an inverse correlation, between almost any type of measure of 5-HT activity and impulsive aggression. This inverse correlation is not reserved for males or females but appears across the genders, though there is some indication that the amount of impulsivity or aggression must be quite severe for our current instruments, probes, and methodologies to determine the presence of a significant difference between cohorts. Certainly further investigations and confirmations of this inverse correlation may lead to more specific pharmacological agents to ameliorate or even reverse an individual's propensity to impulsivity and aggression; in addition, these most recent DNA findings suggest that perhaps someday we may be able to intervene in a curative fashion at the level of the gene.

Catecholamines: Dopamine and Norepinephrine

The study of norepinephrine (NE) and dopamine (DA) in personality disorder has not received the same amount of attention as 5-HT. Although indexes of all three of these neurotransmitters are often investigated simultaneously, typically the findings of relevance, especially in the population with personality disorders, have focused on 5-HT.

Catecholamines in General

Before discussing findings that specifically relate to DA or NE, we review studies that examined the behavioral responses to agents that activate both DA and NE systems.

Based on the hypothesis that subjects with borderline and

schizotypal personality disorders might show different mood and cognitive or perceptual responses to DA or NE stimulants, Schulz et al. (1985) administered, in a controlled setting, acute doses of amphetamine to a series of subjects with personality disorders and then carefully assessed their responses over a period of hours. They reported that eight subjects with borderline personality disorder had greater behavioral sensitivity to an amphetamine administration challenge because these subjects demonstrated an increase in clinician-rated well-being (i.e., the patients reported that they felt much better) as well as an increase in global psychopathology. It is important to note that half of the subjects, compared to none of the normal volunteers, were rated as transiently psychotic during the amphetamine challenge session. In a replication study involving 16 subjects, Schulz et al. (1988) reported that global worsening after administration of amphetamines was typical of subjects with both (comorbid) borderline and schizotypal personality disorder, and global improvement was typical of borderline subjects without comorbid schizotypal personality disorder (thus explaining the inherent contradiction wherein they were rated as having increased well-being while also having increased global psychopathology). These data suggest that there are important biological differences among subjects with borderline personality disorders as a function of comorbid schizotypy. Amphetamine is known to elevate dopamine levels. Elevation of dopaminergic function in subjects with schizotypal personality disorder (Siever et al. 1991, 1993), as will be elaborated on in a later section and in Chapter 2, may contribute to this adverse behavioral response to amphetamines in subjects with comorbid schizotypy.

Dopamine

Studies involving assessments of dopamine function in personality disorder fall into two main areas: schizotypy and aggression.

Two studies support the hypothesis that DA function is directly related to schizotypy. One study reported higher CSF homovanillic acid (HVA—a dopamine metabolite) concentrations in 11 subjects with schizotypal personality disorder (SPD) when compared with 6 healthy volunteer controls (Siever et al. 1993). In addition, the number of psychotic-like schizotypal symptoms correlated positively with CSF HVA concentration ($r = .61$, $P = .007$) in a combined group of 18 subjects with schizotypal and nonschizotypal personality disorders. No correlation existed between non-psychotic-like schizotypal symptoms and CSF HVA concentration. Another study examined plasma HVA concentrations in 10 schizotypal and 14 nonschizotypal subjects; the results of this study revealed a significant elevation in plasma HVA levels in the subjects with SPD (Siever et al. 1991). As with CSF HVA concentration, plasma HVA concentration was found to correlate positively with psychotic-like ($r = .59$, $P = .002$) but not non-psychotic-like ($r = .11$, $P = $ NS) schizotypal symptoms. These data provide preliminary evidence that DA function may be higher in schizotypal subjects and that higher dopamine function may covary with the psychotic-like symptoms (i.e., suspiciousness, ideas of reference, recurrent illusions, and magical thinking) of schizotypal personality, symptoms that may also respond to treatment with low-dose neuroleptics in selected subjects (Coccaro and Siever 1995). This finding makes sense if one considers that schizotypal personality disorder frequently appears in families with schizophrenia, and some consider schizotypal personality disorder to be a *forme fruste* of schizophrenia (Siever and Davis 1991).

Evidence for a role of DA in human aggression is limited. Some studies demonstrate no relationship between CSF HVA concentration and aggression (Brown et al. 1979; Virkkunen et al. 1987), whereas other studies suggest an inverse relationship between these variables. Among the studies that show a relationship, Linnoila et al. (1983) reported a reduction in CSF HVA level in antisocial, though not explosive, impulsive violent offenders, and Virkkunen et al. (1989) reported that recidivist violent offenders had lower CSF HVA concentrations than nonrecidivist violent offender controls. It is of note that in each of these studies a strong inverse relationship between CSF 5-HIAA concentration and the aggression variable was also reported. Given the widely acknowledged observation that CSF 5-HIAA and CSF HVA concentrations are strongly intercorrelated, it is possible that findings with CSF HVA may be related to similar findings with CSF 5-HIAA concentration. In fact, Agren et al. (1986) have argued that CSF 5-HIAA "drives" CSF HVA. If so, a specific assessment of CSF HVA level may not be made unless the effect of CSF 5-HIAA concentration is accounted for. Although this statistical adjustment has not been made in published studies as of this time, we have found a significant inverse relationship between CSF HVA level, when adjusted for CSF 5-HIAA, and a life history of aggression in both male and female subjects with personality disorders. Given that animal studies suggest a direct relationship between DA function and aggression (Coccaro 1996), it is possible that an inverse relationship between CSF HVA concentration and aggression indirectly reflects the positive relationship between postsynaptic DA receptor sensitivity and aggression or arousal, which in turn can increase the likelihood of aggression given the proper circumstances. In this regard, it is noteworthy that a strong positive relationship between positive emotionality and prolactin response to DA receptor agents has been reported in nonpsychiatric subjects (DePue et al. 1994). Thus, while behavioral correlates are certainly related to increases or decreases in dopamine, the amount of work undertaken in this area is scant. This latter fact, as well as the strong intercorrelation between CSF 5-HIAA and CSF HVA, make any findings at this point quite preliminary.

Norepinephrine

Studies involving behavioral assessments of NE function in personality disorder have largely been in the area of aggression as well. As with DA, animal studies suggest a direct relationship between NE function and aggression (Coccaro 1996). Brown et al. (1979) reported a positive correlation between CSF 3-methoxy-4-hydroxyphenylglycol (MHPG—a NE metabolite) concentrations and a life history of aggression in 12 male subjects with personality disorders. Despite this correlation, however, a multiple regression that included CSF 5-HIAA revealed that CSF 5-HIAA accounted for 80% of the variance in aggression scores. According to these results, then, the influence of NE on aggression appeared to be small. In support of at least some role for NE in impulsivity or aggression, Siever and Trestman (1993) reported that plasma NE was modestly, but positively, correlated with self-reported impulsivity in male subjects with personality disorders. In contrast to these studies, however, Virkkunen et al. (1987) reported a significant reduction in CSF MHPG concentration in violent offenders. Recently, we have found a significant reduction in plasma free MHPG in male subjects with personality disorders when compared with normal volunteers. Within the personality disorder group, subjects with borderline personality disorder had lower plasma free MHPG when compared with their nonborderline controls. In addition, there was a modest, but significant, inverse correlation between plasma free MHPG and life history of aggression across all subjects with personality disorders.

NE pharmacological challenge studies in subjects with personality disorders have been limited. Coccaro et al. (1991) reported a positive correlation between the growth hormone response to the α_2 NE agonist clonidine and self-reported irritability (which is thought to be a correlate of aggression) in a small sample of male subjects with personality disorders and healthy volunteers. Together with our findings of an inverse relationship between plasma free MHPG and aggression, it is possible that there may be variable dysregulation of presynaptic (i.e., reflected by plasma free MHPG) and postsynaptic (i.e., reflected by the growth hormone response to clonidine) NE function in subjects with personality disorders who have prominent histories of aggression.

Similar to the issue raised earlier with DA, we can only conclude that although behavioral correlates are certainly related to increases or decreases in NE, much more work needs to be done in this area. Hopefully more sophisticated probes and newer pharmacological challenge studies may eventually clarify the roles that each of these two neurotransmitters play in behavior.

Other Neurotransmitters: Acetylcholine and Vasopressin

Investigations of acetylcholine function, particularly with personality disorders, have been limited to one study. Because enhanced acetylcholine sensitivity has been implicated in affective disorders, it is possible that this neurotransmitter may contribute to the heightened affective sensitivity of selected subjects with personality disorders such as those with borderline personality disorder. Steinberg et al. (1997) examined the behavioral response to acute infusions of the acetylcholinesterase inhibitor physostigmine in 10 subjects with borderline personality disorder, 24 subjects without borderline personality disorder, and 11 healthy volunteers. In this study, subjects with borderline personality disorder reported greater self-rated depression scores than the nonborderline or healthy volunteer cohorts. Peak physostigmine-induced depression scores correlated positively with the number of affective instability ($r = .45$, $P < .01$), but not with the number of impulsive aggressive ($r = .08$, $P =$ NS), borderline personality traits. This finding suggests that physostigmine-induced dysphoria was a specific correlate of affective instability and not of other borderline personality disorder traits. Accordingly, these data suggest that the trait of affective lability in subjects with borderline personality disorder may be mediated, in part, by a heightened sensitivity to acetylcholine.

Only one study of central vasopressin activity has been performed in subjects with personality disorders. Animal studies in lower mammals suggest a positive relationship between central vasopressin and aggression (Ferris and Delville 1994). In our laboratory we have found a significant positive correlation between CSF vasopressin concentrations and a life history of aggression, and of aggression against persons in particular. Most importantly, this relationship was present even after accounting for a separate relationship between aggression and 5-HT levels (Coccaro et al. 1996e).

Thus, unlike the studies with the three neurotransmitters described previously—5-HT, DA, and NE—acetylcholine does not appear to correlate with impulsivity or aggression. Rather, it appears to be related to affective lability, certainly a quality found in many patients with personality disorders, especially those in the dramatic cluster (cluster B). Hopefully, further work in this area will continue to shed light on the role of acetylcholine in this troubling aspect of the behavior of patients with personality disorders.

Conclusions

CNS neurotransmitters clearly have a role in modulating selected personality dimensional traits in subjects with personality disorders. Based on the present data that have accumulated, 5-HT (i.e., serotonin) has an important, though not necessarily unique, role in aggression or impulsive aggression as behaviorally expressed by subjects with personality disorders. Dopamine plays an important role in the positive schizotypal symptoms that refer to cognitive or perceptual distortions and may have a contributory role in aggression as well. Norepinephrine and vasopressin may also be involved in aggression, and acetylcholine may influence underlying affective sensitivity or lability.

Of course all of these associations are merely simplifications of the results of data from a variety of studies using a variety of methodologies among heterogeneous groups of subjects. Further research is required to deepen our understanding of the role of central neurotransmitter function in subjects with personality disorders. Only with this understanding can we develop selective and effective primary, or adjunctive, pharmacological treatments for the more severe and socially disruptive manifestations of personality disorders.

References

Agren H, Mefford IN, Rudorfer MV, et al: Interacting neurotransmitter systems: a non-experimental approach to the 5-HIAA–HVA correlation in human CSF. J Psychiatr Res 20:175–193, 1986

American Psychiatric Association: Diagnostic and Statistical Manual of Mental Disorders, 2nd Edition. Washington, DC, American Psychiatric Association, 1968

American Psychiatric Association: Diagnostic and Statistical Manual of Mental Disorders, 3rd Edition. Washington, DC, American Psychiatric Association, 1980

Asberg M, Traksman L, Thoren P: 5-HIAA in the cerebrospinal fluid: a biochemical suicide predictor? Arch Gen Psychiatry 33:1193–1197, 1976

Bernstein DP, Handlesman L: The neurobiology of substance abuse and personality disorders, in Neuropsychiatry of Personality Disorders. Edited by Ratey JJ. Cambridge, MA, Blackwell Scientific, 1995, pp 120–148

Biegon A, Grinspoon A, Blumenfeld B, et al: Increased serotonin 5-HT$_2$ receptor binding on blood platelets of suicidal men. Psychopharmacology 100:165–167, 1990

Birmaher B, Stanley M, Greenhill L, et al: Platelet imipramine binding in children and adolescents with impulsive behavior. J Am Acad Child Adolesc Psychiatry 29:914–918, 1990

Brown GL, Goodwin FK, Ballenger JC, et al: Aggression in humans correlates with cerebrospinal fluid amine metabolites. Psychiatry Res 1:131–139, 1979

Brown GL, Ebert MH, Goyer PF, et al: Aggression, suicide, and serotonin: relationships to CSF amine metabolites. Am J Psychiatry 139:741–746, 1982

Coccaro EF: Neurotransmitter correlates of impulsive aggression in humans. Ann N Y Acad Sci 794:82–89, 1996

Coccaro EF, Kavoussi RJ: The neuropsychopharmacologic challenge in biological psychiatry. Clin Chem 40:319–327, 1994

Coccaro EF, Siever LJ: The neuropsychopharmacology of personality disorder, in Psychopharmacology: The Fourth Generation of Progress. Edited by Bloom F, Kupfer D. New York, Raven, 1995

Coccaro EF, Siever LJ, Klar HM, et al: Serotonergic studies in affective and personality disorders: correlates with suicidal and impulsive aggressive behavior. Arch Gen Psychiatry 46:587–599, 1989

Coccaro EF, Gabriel S, Siever LJ: Buspirone challenge: preliminary evidence for a role for 5-HT-1a receptors in impulsive aggressive behavior in humans. Psychopharmacol Bull 26:393–405, 1990

Coccaro EF, Lawrence T, Trestman R, et al: Growth hormone responses to intravenous clonidine challenge correlates with behavioral irritability in psychiatric patients and in healthy volunteers. Psychiatry Res 39:129–139, 1991

Coccaro EF, Kavoussi RJ, Hauger RL: Physiologic responses to d-fenfluramine and ipsapirone challenge correlate with indices of aggression in males with personality disorder. Int Clin Psychopharmacol 10:177–180, 1995

Coccaro EF, Kavoussi RJ, Berman ME, et al: Relationship of prolactin response to d-fenfluramine to behavioral and questionnaire assessments of aggression in personality disordered males. Biol Psychiatry 40:157–164, 1996a

Coccaro EF, Kavoussi RJ, Oakes M, et al: Amesergide completely blocks the prolactin response to d-fenfluramine in healthy male subjects. Psychopharmacology 126:24–30, 1996b

Coccaro EF, Kavoussi RJ, Cooper TB, et al: 5-HT-3 receptor antagonism by ondansetron does not attenuate the prolactin response to d-fenfluramine challenge in healthy male subjects. Psychopharmacology 127:108–112, 1996c

Coccaro EF, Kavoussi RJ, Sheline YI, et al: Impulsive aggression in personality disorder: correlates with ^{3}H-paroxetine binding in the platelet. Arch Gen Psychiatry 53:531–536, 1996d

Coccaro EF, Kavoussi RJ, Hauger RL, et al: CSF vasopressin: correlates with indices of aggression and serotonin function in personality disordered subjects. Abstracts of the 35th Annual Meeting of the American College of Neuropsychopharmacology, San Juan, Puerto Rico, 1996e, p 243

Coccaro EF, Kavoussi RJ, Cooper TB, et al: Central serotonin and aggression: inverse relationship with prolactin response to d-fenfluramine, but not with CSF 5-HIAA concentration in human subjects. Am J Psychiatry 154:1430–1435, 1997a

Coccaro EF, Kavoussi RJ, Sheline YI, et al: Impulsive aggression in personality disorder: correlates with ^{125}I-LSD binding in the platelet. Neuropsychopharmacology 16:211–216, 1997b

Coccaro EF, Kavoussi RJ, Trestman RL, et al: Serotonin function in personality and mood disorder: intercorrelations among central indices and aggressiveness. Psychiatry Res (in press)

Cook EH, Fletcher KE, Wainwright M, et al: Primary structure of the human platelet serotonin 5-HT-2a receptor: identity with frontal cortex serotonin 5-HT-2a receptor. J Neurochem 63:465–469, 1994

DePue RA, Luciana M, Arbisi P, et al: Dopamine and the structure of personality: relation of agonist-induced dopamine activity to positive emotionality. J Pers Soc Psychol 67:485–498, 1994

Ferris CF, Delville Y: Vasopressin and serotonin interactions in the control of agonistic behavior. Psychoneuroendocrinology 19:593–601, 1994

Fishbein DH, Lozovsky D, Jaffe JH: Impulsivity, aggression, and neuroendocrine responses to serotonergic stimulation in substance abusers. Biol Psychiatry 25:1049–1066, 1989

Gardner DL, Lucas PB, Cowdry RW: CSF metabolites in borderline personality disorder compared with normal controls. Biol Psychiatry 28:247–254, 1990

Goodall EM, Cowan PJ, Franklin M, et al: Ritanserin attenuates anorectic, endocrine, and thermal responses to *d*-fenfluramine in human volunteers. Psychopharmacology 112:461–466, 1993

Handlesman L, Holloway K, Kahn RS, et al: Hostility is associated with a low prolactin response to meta-chlorophenylpiperazine in abstinent alcoholics. Alcohol Clin Exp Res 20:824–829, 1996

Hathaway SR, McKinley JC: Minnesota Multiphasic Personality Inventory. Minneapolis, MN, University of Minnesota, 1943

Hollander E, Stein D, DeCaria CM, et al: Serotonergic sensitivity in borderline personality disorder: preliminary findings. Am J Psychiatry 151:277–280, 1994

Lesch K-P, Wolozin BL, Murphy DL, et al: Primary structure of the human platelet serotonin uptake site: identity with the brain serotonin transporter. J Neurochem 60:2319–2322, 1993

Linnoila M, Virkkunen M, Scheinin M, et al: Low cerebrospinal fluid 5-hydroxyindoleacetic acid concentration differentiates impulsive from nonimpulsive violent behavior. Life Sci 33:2609–2614, 1983

Mann JJ, McBride PA, Anderson GM, et al: Platelet and whole blood serotonin content in depressed inpatients: correlations with acute and life-time psychopathology. Biol Psychiatry 32:243–257, 1992

Marazziti D, Rotondo A, Presta S, et al: Role of serotonin in human aggressive behavior. Aggressive Behavior 9:347–353, 1993

McBride PA, Brown RP, DeMeo M, et al: The relationship of platelet 5-HT-2 receptor indices to major depressive disorder, personality trait, and suicidal behavior. Biol Psychiatry 35:295–308, 1994

Meltzer HY, Maes M: Pindolol pretreatment blocks stimulation by meta-chlorophenylpiperazine of prolactin but not cortisol secretion in normal men. Psychiatry Res 58:89–98, 1995

Moss HB, Yao JK, Panzak GL: Serotonergic responsivity and behavioral dimensions in antisocial personality disorder with substance abuse. Biol Psychiatry 28:325–338, 1990

Murphy DL, Mellow AM, Sunderland T, et al: Strategies for the study of serotonin in humans, in Serotonin in Major Psychiatric Disorders. Edited by Coccaro EF, Murphy DL. Washington, DC, American Psychiatric Press, 1990, pp 3–25

New AS, Trestman RL, Mitroupoulou V, et al: Serotonergic function and self-injurious behavior in personality disorder patients. Psychiatry Res 69:17–26, 1997

New AS, Gelernter J, Yovell Y, et al: Tryptophan hydroxylase genotype is associated with impulsive aggression measures: a preliminary study. Am J Hum Genet (in press)

Nielsen DA, Goldman D, Virkkunen M, et al: Suicidality and

5-hydroxyindoleacetic acid concentration associated with a tryptophan hydroxylase polymorphism. Arch Gen Psychiatry 51:34–38, 1994

O'Keane V, Moloney E, O'Neill H, et al: Blunted prolactin responses to d-fenfluramine in sociopathy: evidence for subsensitivity of central serotonergic function. Br J Psychiatry 160:643–646, 1992

Pandey GN, Pandey SC, Dwivedi Y, et al: Platelet serotonin-2a receptors: a potential biological marker for suicidal behavior. Am J Psychiatry 152:850–855, 1995

Park SBG, Cowen PJ: Effect of pindolol on the prolactin response to d-fenfluramine. Psychopharmacology 118:471–474, 1995

Plomin R, Owen MJ, McGuffin P: The genetic basis of complex human behaviors. Science 264:1733–1739, 1994

Schulz SC, Schulz PM, Dommisse C, et al: Amphetamine response in borderline patients. Psychiatry Res 15:97–108, 1985

Schulz SC, Cornelius J, Schulz PM, et al: The amphetamine challenge test in patients with borderline personality disorder. Am J Psychiatry 145:809–814, 1988

Seibyl JP, Krystal JH, Price LH, et al: Effects of ritanserin on the behavioral, neuroendocrine, and cardiovascular response to meta-chlorophenylpiperazine in healthy human subjects. Psychiatry Res 38:227–236, 1991

Siever LJ, Davis KL: A psychobiological perspective on the personality disorders. Am J Psychiatry 148:1647–1658, 1991

Siever L, Trestman RL: The serotonin system and aggressive personality disorder. Int Clin Psychopharmacol 8(suppl 2):33–39, 1993

Siever LJ, Amin F, Coccaro EF, et al: Plasma homovanillic acid in schizotypal personality disorder. Am J Psychiatry 148:1246–1248, 1991

Siever LJ, Amin F, Coccaro EF, et al: CSF homovanillic acid in schizotypal personality disorder. Am J Psychiatry 150:149–151, 1993

Simansky KJ, Schechter LE: Properties of some 1-arylpiperazines as antagonists of stereotyped behaviors mediated by central serotonergic receptors in rodents. J Pharmacol Exp Ther 247:1073–1081, 1988

Simeon D, Stanley B, Frances A, et al: Self-mutilation in personality disorders: psychological and biological correlates. Am J Psychiatry 149:221–226, 1992

Stanley M, Ttaksman-Bendz L, Dorovini-Zis K: Correlations between aminergic metabolites simultaneously obtained from human CSF and brain. Life Sci 37:1279–1286, 1985

Stein DJ, Trestman RL, Mitroupoulou V, et al: Impulsivity and serotonergic function in compulsive personality disorder. J Neuropsychiatry Clin Neurosci 8:393–398, 1996

Steinberg BJ, Trestman R, Mitroupoulou V, et al: Depressive response to physostigmine challenge in borderline personality disorder patients. Neuropsychopharmacology 17:264–273, 1997

Stoff DM, Pollock L, Vitiello B, et al: Reduction of 3-H-imipramine binding sites on platelets of conduct disordered children. Neuropsychopharmacology 1:55–62, 1987

Valzelli L: Psychobiology of Aggression and Violence. New York, Raven, 1980

Virkkunen M, Nuutila A, Goodwin FK, et al: Cerebrospinal fluid monoamine metabolite levels in male arsonists. Arch Gen Psychiatry 44:241–247, 1987

Virkkunen M, DeJong J, Bartko J, et al: Relationship of psychobiological variables to recidivism in violent offenders and impulsive fire setters. Arch Gen Psychiatry 46:600–603, 1989

Chapter 2

New Biological Research Strategies for Personality Disorders

Larry J. Siever, M.D., Antonia S. New, M.D., Richelle Kirrane, M.D., Sherie Novotny, M.D., Harold Koenigsberg, M.D., and Robert Grossman, M.D.

The study of the neurobiology of personality disorders represents a relatively recent field of inquiry when compared with biologically based investigations of the Axis I disorders. Initial studies borrowed techniques and specific measures that have been applied to Axis I disorders such as schizophrenia or depression; these studies included measures of rapid eye movement (REM) latency or responses to the dexamethasone suppression test and applied them to the Axis II disorders (Weston and Siever 1993). From that point, the studies progressed to more sophisticated examinations of neurotransmitter metabolites or neuroendocrine responses to neurotransmitter challenges as well as to electrophysiologic or psychophysiologic tasks. More recently, the field has seen the emergence of new strategies that lend themselves particularly to the study of personality disorders while utilizing the latest in clinical neuroscience techniques. These studies target behavioral dimensions that lie at the core of the personality disorders and capitalize on naturalistic variations in such dimensions as impulsivity, affective instability, or cognitive dysfunction to characterize antecedent psychosocial variables such as trauma, neuroanatomic circuits as revealed by imaging, pharmacological interventions for cognitive dysfunction, and predisposing candidate genes. These areas are reviewed in the context of their implications for ongoing personality disorder research.

Strategies to Assess Sequelae of Trauma

Background

Human behavior is a complex product, influenced by genetic as well as environmental factors. Some of the most powerful environmental events are psychological stresses such as sexual abuse, physical abuse, emotional neglect, and physical neglect. As opposed to trauma occurring in other psychiatric populations, there is evidence that in patients with personality disorders, trauma has often been experienced during childhood or latency (Herman et al. 1989; Zanarini et al. 1989), frequently involves the patient's caregivers (Paris and Zweig-Frank 1992), and is notable for its marked severity and lengthy duration (Herman et al. 1989). If such abuse occurs during a developmental period of increased physiological vulnerability, there may be a greater chance that it will result in long-term neurobiological and neuroendocrine alterations in these individuals.

Investigators have forwarded and debated the provocative conceptualization of borderline personality disorder (BPD) as a type of trauma-related disorder resulting from chronic early abuse (Gunderson and Sabo 1993; Herman et al. 1989). Indeed, it has been suggested that BPD is actually a variant of posttraumatic stress disorder (PTSD). Herman (1992) proposed using the term *complex PTSD* to denote the syndrome of dissociative symptoms, identity diffusion, somatization, and impulsivity or affective instability seen in adult survivors of chronic childhood abuse. BPD criteria have been found to be directly correlated with frequency of sexual abuse (New et al. 1996). It is clear, however, that not all BPD subjects have experienced abuse, and, of those who have, classical PTSD symptoms do not necessarily ensue. Biologically comparing BPD subjects with abused and PTSD subjects could provide useful information in the role played by abuse in BPD neurobiology, as well as in the relationship between BPD and PTSD.

The neurobiology of trauma centers on the hypothalamic-pituitary-adrenal (HPA) axis, which is the central neuroendocrine stress-response regulator. The well-known dexamethasone suppression test (DST) is designed to test HPA axis feedback mechanisms. This test is performed by administering 1.0 mg of dexamethasone (a synthetic steroid) and then measuring how much the body suppresses endogenous cortisol production. In healthy nonpsychiatric subjects, the exogenous dexamethasone greatly diminishes endogenous cortisol. Other HPA axis measures include concentration of urinary cortisol, amount of cortisol excreted in the urine over 24 hours, and round-the-clock sampling of plasma cortisol through intravenous cannula, with later chronobiological analysis. A newer technique involves utilizing a cytosolic radioligand–binding assay to measure the density of plasma lymphocyte glucocorticoid receptors (GRs) as an index of central neuronal GR density. GRs are necessary for translocation of steroid into the nucleus for genomic effects; they also provide feedback control over HPA activity at the level of the pituitary.

Utilization of these techniques with various modifications has greatly clarified HPA axis activity in the prototypical stress-induced psychiatric disorder, namely, PTSD. PTSD subjects, as compared with traumatized subjects without PTSD, have decreased urinary cortisol excretion, lower baseline levels of plasma cortisol, and increased density of GRs on peripheral lymphocytes (Yehuda 1998). Chronobiological analysis revealed that PTSD subjects had a greater signal to noise ratio (increased feedback sensitivity) and a decreased cortisol mesor (average cortisol level over 24 hours) as compared with subjects with major depressive disorder (MDD) and normal controls (Yehuda 1998). It is as if the HPA axis were adjusted to a greater sensitivity setting with a lower basal cortisol, heightened sensitivity to feedback regulation, and greater responsiveness.

These HPA axis findings in PTSD are opposite to those found in MDD—that is, MDD is associated with increased urinary cortisol excretion, decreased density of lymphocyte GRs (Yehuda 1998), and decreased signal to noise ratio in basal cortisol levels subjected to 24-hour chronobiological analysis (Yehuda 1998). The most widely known HPA axis finding in psychiatry is that approximately 40% of MDD subjects have DST nonsuppression. MDD subjects therefore have increased basal cortisol levels and

GR downregulation accompanied by decreased HPA axis negative feedback sensitivity. In patients with MDD, then, there is minimal feedback inhibition and little responsiveness to the environment.

In further exploration of the differences between HPA axis findings in PTSD and MDD, the DST was modified to change it from an instrument sensitive for the detection of *decreased* negative feedback (nonsuppression, as in MDD) to one sensitive to *increased* negative feedback, or hypersuppression. This change was made by decreasing the dexamethasone dose to 0.5 mg or 0.25 mg. Utilizing this low-dose DST (LD-DST), subjects with PTSD were found to have an enhanced suppression of cortisol compared with both combat-exposed veterans without PTSD and normal controls (Yehuda 1998). Using a 0.25-mg dose of dexamethasone, cortisol hypersuppression was found to be significantly associated with the severity of PTSD symptoms (Yehuda 1998). These findings indicate that subjects with PTSD have decreased baseline cortisol levels and GR downregulation accompanied by increased HPA axis negative feedback sensitivity (Yehuda 1998). PTSD subjects therefore have increased basal cortisol levels and GR downregulation accompanied by decreased HPA axis negative feedback sensitivity. Many of these studies utilized control subjects who sustained identical traumas but who did not develop PTSD. It can therefore be stated that in the subjects studied, these HPA axis alterations were associated not with trauma in general but specifically with PTSD.

As a means to understand neuroendocrine function in BPD and other personality disorders in relation to PTSD and abuse history, the LD-DST and GR analyses have begun to be employed in subjects with personality disorders (Grossman et al. 1997). If BPD was simply a variant of depression, as has been proposed (Akiskal 1981), the DST results would resemble those of patients with MDD; however, if BPD was more closely related to PTSD, BPD patients would have profiles more closely related to those of PTSD patients. In a pilot study of 14 subjects without psychiatric disorders and without history of abuse, 9 subjects with history of abuse and with at least one personality disorder, and 14 veterans with PTSD, HPA axis assessments were performed.

HPA axis measures included baseline cortisol and plasma lymphocyte GR number and percentage cortisol suppression following the administration of 0.5 mg of dexamethasone. All subjects were medically healthy and had not taken any medications for a minimum of 2 weeks.

Subjects with personality disorders had the lowest basal cortisol level of all three groups. They still displayed marked sensitivity to cortisol suppression by dexamethasone. Of the three subjects with personality disorders who were not LD-DST hypersuppressors, two had comorbid MDD. Only one of the six cortisol hypersuppressors had comorbid MDD.

Basal GR number per lymphocyte in subjects with personality disorders was lower than the basal GR number in subjects with PTSD. Of the subjects with personality disorders, however, the two patients with comorbid PTSD had an average basal GR number similar to that of the "pure" PTSD patients.

Taken together, subjects with personality disorders but without comorbid MDD or PTSD appear to present with a novel pattern of HPA axis activity, namely, decreased basal cortisol and cortisol hypersuppression associated with abuse and increased lymphocyte GR density that may be associated with PTSD symptomatology. Decreased basal cortisol and cortisol hypersuppression may be a trait marker for personality disorders, whereas decreased GR number may be a state measure associated with PTSD (Grossman et al. 1997; R. Grossman and R. Yehuda unpublished data, October 1996). Thus, patients with personality disorders do not demonstrate the profiles of either MDD or PTSD, although their patterns are more closely related to the PTSD than the MDD pattern. Why might subjects with personality disorders, the majority having BPD, display the seemingly novel combination of HPA axis findings?

Serotonergic pathways are one of the strongest modulators of the HPA axis. Therefore, altered serotonergic functioning as associated with impulsive aggressive behavior in subjects with personality disorders may alter modulation and reactivity of the HPA axis in these subjects.

The majority of studies on HPA-serotonin interaction are preclinical. Early handling of rat pups has been found to permanently increase hippocampal GRs (Meaney et al. 1989), but this phenomenon could be induced only during a narrow developmental period. This finding may be of particular relevance to subjects with personality disorders whose trauma tends to be of a chronic nature and occurs during childhood. Serotonergic pathways appear to play a permissive role since both chemical and physical lesions of serotonergic pathways leading to the hippocampus prevent this GR upregulation (Mitchell et al. 1990). Normal modulation of the HPA axis in relation to trauma appears to require intact serotonergic functioning. In vitro, 5-hydroxytryptamine (5-HT) stimulation of cultured hippocampal neurons increases GR density (Mitchell et al. 1990), and antidepressants that increase serotonergic functioning increase GR mRNA and GR number. Conversely, the selective 5-HT neurotoxin parachloroamphetamine has been found to acutely decrease hippocampal glucocorticoid receptors (Novotny and Lowry 1995). Decreased serotonergic stimulation of 5-HT$_{1a}$ receptors results in decreased release of cortisol-releasing hormone (CRH), adrenocorticotropin hormone (ACTH), and corticosterone or cortisol.

In a reciprocal fashion, the HPA axis has clear effects on serotonergic activity. Increasing cortisol levels results in increased tryptophan hydroxylase activity (the rate limiting enzyme in the formation of serotonin) (Azmitia et al. 1993), increased levels of tryptophan 2,3-dioxygenase (the rate limiting enzyme in the catabolism of tryptophan), and increased firing of serotonergic neurons in the dorsal and median raphe nuclei. Increasing corticosterone levels and activation of GRs result in inhibition of both transcription (Meijer and de Kloet 1994) and translation of the 5-HT$_{1a}$ receptor gene. Increased corticosterone levels also results in greater 5-HT$_{1a}$–induced hyperpolarization (Laaris et al. 1995). Thus, cortisol has both inhibitory and facilitatory roles on serotonergic activity both pre- and postsynaptically at 5-HT$_{1a}$ receptors. Clinical data have demonstrated that prolactin response to serotonergic probes is inversely correlated with basal cortisol level in subjects with MDD and more recently in those with bipolar disorder. HPA axis–serotonergic interactions appear to be present in our pilot data in subjects with personality disorders.

We have compared HPA axis measures and the prolactin response to fenfluramine challenge (ΔPRL FEN) in subjects with personality disorders in order to assess the HPA-serotonergic interactions. In subjects with personality disorders, basal cortisol level had a negative correlation with ΔPRL FEN ($r = -.82$, $N = 7$, $P = .023$), which is in agreement with published data from subjects with MDD and bipolar disorder (high basal cortisol concentration is associated with blunted serotonergic response). Lymphocyte GR number at basal also appears to be negatively correlated with ΔPRL FEN ($r = -.48$, $N = 7$, $P = .271$) (high basal GR number is associated with blunted serotonergic response). Both increased cortisol levels and GR numbers would be hypothesized to result in increased total cortisol "activity" and therefore decreased serotonergic reactivity to challenge. To the extent that GR upregulation occurs, as in individuals exposed to severe abuse and with PTSD symptomatology, this may further serve to decrease serotonergic function and may account for these biological relationships in the most traumatized subjects. Further, decreased serotonergic functioning in individuals with impulsive aggressive personality disorder may alter vulnerability to traumatic stressors.

Implications

In summary, the instruments of the LD-DST and GR analysis, along with other HPA axis measures, can be useful in the process of understanding the role of trauma in personality disorders and the relationship between personality disorders (particularly BPD) and PTSD. The relationship among trauma, PTSD, and BPD has received lively debate, yet our preliminary studies constitute the first attempt to address this question neurobiologically. Further, decreased serotonergic activity in subjects with personality disorders may play an important role in the modulation of HPA axis adaptability or alterations as related to abuse and PTSD. Associations among trauma history, symptomatology (both personality disorder and PTSD), and neurobiological measures can be explored through these means. These preliminary studies suggest that investigating the neuroendocrine axis as related to trauma and depression will be an important aspect in understanding the psychobiology of the personality disorders.

Neuroimaging Strategies

Neuroimaging methodologies offer the opportunity to identify brain structural alterations that may be associated with personality disorder dimensions (such as cognitive disorganization or social withdrawal) and functionally assess brain activity via measurements of blood flow or metabolic activity. Specific issues related to cognitive dysfunction in schizophrenia spectrum personality disorders are discussed in the later section on cognitive neuropsychology; in this section we focus on functional imaging studies that provide an opportunity to identify key brain networks involved in the pathophysiology of impulsivity and affective instability in disorders such as BPD. Both baseline resting studies that can characterize alterations in activity associated with these dimensions and studies of responses to pharmacological perturbations of a system such as the serotonergic system that may modify these key circuits will be explored.

Technologies for visualizing the structure and functioning of the living brain have developed over the last several years and place us at the threshold of a deeper understanding of the relationship between psychiatric disorders and dysfunctional brain activity. The advent of computed tomography (CT) and magnetic resonance imaging (MRI) have enabled us to observe brain structures with better spatial resolution and sharper definition between gray and white matter. Positron-emission tomography (PET), single photon emission computed tomography (SPECT), and functional magnetic resonance imaging (fMRI) enable us to visualize regional patterns of activation within the working brain. Magnetic resonance spectroscopy (MRS), the newest of the techniques, will allow us to localize specific neurochemical processes within the functioning brain. These methods already have generated important new hypotheses about the psychobiology of schizophrenia, the major affective disorders, obsessive-compulsive disorder, panic disorder, PTSD, and the dementias. As yet, they have only begun to be applied to the personality disorders.

These techniques are well suited to examining a number of important questions about the personality disorders. The extent to which neurobiology plays a role in personality functioning, the relationship between normal personality traits and personality disorder, the choice of a categorical versus dimensional model for classifying the personality disorders, the relationship between Axis II and phenomenologically related Axis I disorders, and the biological mechanisms underlying personality dysfunction may all be addressed using neuroimaging methods.

The choice of which imaging technique to use for a particular research study is determined by a number of factors. Methods with high spatial resolution and good discrimination between gray and white matter are necessary for anatomical localization of small structures. High temporal resolution is necessary for examining task-related changes in brain activation. Studies in which it is important to localize brain activity to specific anatomic structures require techniques that permit the coregistration of high-resolution functional and anatomic images. The length of time required for image acquisition may constrain the number of brain regions that can be studied or the number of manipulations that can be carried out without overtaxing the subject. Some techniques require radioisotopes with such short half-lives that proximity to a cyclotron is necessary. Cumulative radiation dosage can limit repeated procedures in PET and SPECT. Before considering specific research strategies for the personality disorders, we briefly review the imaging techniques themselves.

Techniques for Functional Imaging

PET imaging permits visualization of brain activity by locating the distribution of radiolabeled compounds in the brain. It takes advantage of the fact that positrons are annihilated by local electrons within millimeters of their point of emission and that annihilation gives rise to two photons that travel in exactly opposite directions. In PET scanning, the subject's head is positioned within a ring of scintillation counters. Counters diametrically opposite each other on the ring triggered simultaneously indicates a positron emission somewhere along the line connecting the counters. Additional information localizing the source point along this line is obtained by comparing the arrival times of the two photons at the detectors. As coincident counts are accumulated from all of the detectors on the ring, it becomes possible to localize the positron sources and construct an image of the distribution of radioisotope in a slice of brain. Positron-emitting radioisotopes are available for labeling water, deoxyglucose, dopamine D_2 receptor ligands, and opiate receptor ligands. These compounds permit studies of regional cerebral blood flow (rCBF); regional cerebral metabolic rate of glucose (rCMRG), a good measure of local synaptic activity; and D_2 and opiate binding, respectively. More recently, tracers have been developed to study muscarinic receptors and the in vivo metabolism of dopamine and monoamine oxidase. Current PET scans have spatial resolutions of 4–10 mm, with 1–2 mm being a theoretical lower limit (Holcomb et al. 1989). Time resolutions ranging from tens of minutes to less than a minute are possible, depending on the half-life of the radioisotope selected and its retention time in the brain. At present, the radioisotopes that permit fast time resolution afford poorer spatial resolution and vice versa.

SPECT imaging is also based on the localization of radiolabeled compounds. It employs isotopes that emit only a single photon and detects them using a ring array of counters. Without the availability of two 180-degree separated photons to define a line through the brain, SPECT uses narrow lead collimators in front of the detectors to define a line of entry for the photons. Narrowing the collimator improves spatial resolution but reduces the number of counts detectable and lowers the signal to noise ratio. SPECT spatial resolutions are not as high as those obtainable with PET. Radiochemicals are available for SPECT measurement of rCBF and receptor binding.

MRI is based on the release of stored energy in the form of a radio pulse when nuclei with magnetic moments are induced to reverse their orientation in a magnetic field. The strength of this signal depends on the magnetic moment of the nuclei, the proton density in the tissue, the flow velocity of the nuclei, and the homogeneity of the local magnetic field. By varying the timing and sequence of the train of inducing radio signal pulses, it is possible to obtain signals more sensitive to either the proton density of the tissue or the characteristics of the local magnetic field interactions in the neighborhood of the nuclei. One pulse sequence (T_1-weighting) provides excellent definition of anatomic structures and differentiates gray from white matter, whereas a different pulse sequence (T_2-weighting) emphasizes differences between normal and pathological tissue.

Neuronal activity leads to rapid changes in local blood flow and oxygenation. Both of these processes may be detected by MRI scanning without the use of extrinsic contrast agents, the former because flow velocity directly affects MRI signal strength and the latter because of the fortunate coincidence that deoxygenated hemoglobin is a paramagnetic substance. MRI used to image neuronal activity is referred to as fMRI. By selecting the appropriate pulse sequence, one can obtain a blood flow–based fMRI signal or a blood oxygen level–dependent (BOLD) fMRI signal. The latter technique is more commonly used because it requires less a priori information about characteristics of blood flow in the brain. fMRI can achieve spatial resolutions typically of 5–10 mm and time resolutions of seconds (Lee et al. 1996). Using BOLD imaging, regional brain activation has been detected as soon as 3 seconds after a voluntary motor task lasting only half of a second (Bandettini et al. 1995). In addition to good spatial and time resolution, other advantages of fMRI are that it requires no extrinsic contrast agent and there is no radiation exposure. Finally, the same scanning session can be used to obtain an MRI anatomic image that may be readily coregistered with the fMRI images.

Neuronal activity correlating with a particular mental task or stimulus can be measured by presenting the task or stimulus in a repetitive on-off cycle and either subtracting the fMRI images acquired during the off period from those acquired during the on state or correlating the changing fMRI signal at a given pixel with the on-off cycle of the stimulus. Using these methods, fMRI has been utilized to study brain activation during such cognitive tasks as motor control, mental rehearsal of motor tasks, visual processing, speech perception, working memory, and spatial memory.

Studies to Date

Structural Imaging

In studies of schizophrenia, CT and MRI have identified ventricular and possibly sulcal enlargement and decreased temporal lobe volume. In the affective disorders, the most consistent structural finding is of MRI hyperintensities in the subcortical white matter and periventricular regions (Soares and Mann 1997). Thus far, few structural imaging studies of the personality disorders have been carried out. Because of the hypothesized relationship between schizotypal personality disorder (SPD) and schizophrenia, some of the first neuroimaging studies of the personality disorders have looked for the structural features of schizophrenia in schizotypal disorder. Siever (1991) reported enlarged ventricles in patients with schizotypal personality disorder. Raine et al. (1992) found that in a group of nonpatients, high scores on a schizotypal scale were associated with decreased prefrontal area as measured on MRI. Structural imaging studies of small numbers of BPD patients have failed to find ventricular enlargement (Goyer et al. 1994b).

Functional Imaging

Functional imaging methods not only can be applied to search for differences in regional brain activity between normality and the various personality disorders and among the personality disorders themselves but can also identify characteristic patterns of neuronal activity in patients with personality disorders associated with carrying out specific cognitive and emotional tasks. A number of experimental strategies are quite promising. To identify differences in brain functioning between different personality disorders, regional metabolic activity can be compared among diagnostic groups. Because functional neuroimaging is sensitive to the particular cognitive and sensory processing going on in the subject at the time of the study, it is important to standardize what subjects are doing. Some investigators instruct subjects to lie still, relaxing, with eyes closed; others provide a standard cognitive task, such as the visual or auditory continuous performance task (CPT).

One experimental strategy involves studying subjects while they are engaged in a task that is presumed to be specifically affected by their personality disorder. Intrator and co-workers (1997) used SPECT to compare rCBF in a group of psychopathic substance abusers, nonpsychopathic substance abusers, and normal controls engaged in a lexical decision task contrasting the processing of emotional and neutral words. This task was selected because it was hypothesized that psychopathic individuals have a decreased responsivity to the emotional content of language. The investigators found, in fact, that psychopathic and nonpsychopathic individuals displayed different patterns of rCBF in the frontal temporal and medial frontal regions when processing emotional and neutral words.

Affective instability is a pathological personality trait that characterizes patients with BPD. Such patients appear to be especially reactive to emotional stimuli and also show a slower return of their emotional reactions to baseline. Functional neuroimaging could be used to compare the rate of rise and fall, as well as the overall magnitude, of regional brain activation in response to emotional stimuli in affectively unstable patients and controls. We would expect a greater magnitude of activation, possibly a more widely disseminated activation, and a slower return to baseline in BPD patients following an emotional stimulus than in a control population. Such a study has not yet been undertaken, but PET studies of healthy volunteers (George et al. 1995) have identified changes in rCBF in response to mood changes induced by recalling happy or sad events or viewing film clips selected to evoke happiness, sadness, fear, or disgust. With its superior time resolution, fMRI is well suited to studying the time course of emotional activation and return to baseline in borderline patients. Patients with affective instability and normal controls could be challenged with affectively stimulating and neutral photographs while BOLD fMRI images are acquired. Three normal women have been studied by Irwin and colleagues (1996), who found increased activation of the amygdalae bilaterally during the viewing of negative compared with neutral valence photographs.

Functional imaging can also be used to identify changes in brain activation associated with effective treatment. Although this approach has not yet been applied to the study of personality disorders, changes in brain activity following effective psychotherapy, as well as pharmacotherapy, have been documented using neuroimaging techniques. Using PET, Schwartz and colleagues (1996) compared regional glucose metabolic rates in nine patients with obsessive-compulsive disorder before and after 10 weeks of cognitive-behavioral therapy. They reported that therapy responders had significant bilateral decreases in caudate activity compared with nonresponders. In a PET study of patients with major depression treated with sertraline, Buchsbaum et al. (1997) showed that sertraline normalized the rates of metabolic activity in regions characterized by decreased activity in major depression. Moreover, the increase in metabolic rate in the cingulate gyrus correlated with the degree of improvement in depression measured by the Hamilton Rating Scale for Depression (Hamilton 1960). Analogous PET and fMRI studies could be carried out to identify changes in regional activity associated with decreases in impulsive aggression and emotional instability in BPD patients treated with such medications as selective serotonin reuptake inhibitors (SSRIs) and carbamazepine.

Another powerful design combines functional imaging with the use of biological challenge agents. If agents known to activate specific neurotransmitter systems are employed, it is possible to obtain anatomic maps of the activity of these systems in the personality disorders. It has been shown that a blunted prolactin response to the serotonin-releasing or reuptake-blocking agent fenfluramine is correlated with impulsive aggressive behavior, suggesting that serotonin dysregulation may be associated with this behavior. Prolactin response, however, is a measure of serotonergic activity in the hypothalamic-pituitary system and not in brain regions that might mediate impulsive aggression. Functional imaging studies of regional activation in response to a fenfluramine challenge in impulsive aggressive subjects and normal subjects could identify differences in serotonergic activity directly in regions associated with impulsive and aggressive behavior.

From a neuroanatomic viewpoint, the control of aggression and impulsivity has been thought to reside primarily in the frontal cortex since the days of Phineas Gage, the railroad worker who sustained an injury to his frontal cortex in the 1800s and subsequently underwent a radical personality change, with severe increases in his aggressiveness and impulsivity. A recent reconstruction of Gage's wound shows the lesion to be through the anterior and medial aspects of the frontal cortex, bilaterally, but more severe in the left, or dominant, hemisphere (Damasio et al. 1994). Other anecdotal reports of such lesions have noted personality changes, especially in the control of aggression and impulsivity, after injury. More formal studies of violent prisoners and neuropsychiatric patients have shown that frontal cortex impairment has been associated with increased aggression and impulsivity (Heinrichs 1989). One study comparing aggressive psychopathic criminals to depressed ones showed that, although both had lesions in the frontal cortex, the aggressive criminals showed a greater degree of dysfunction on the dominant hemisphere. Another study showed that irritability and angry outbursts were associated with damage to the orbital frontal lobes in neurological patients. Overall, these studies suggest that the orbital frontal cortex appears to be involved in the inhibition of aggression and impulsivity. Other studies, including animal lesioning studies, have associated these traits with areas in the temporal lobes and amygdala; however, these studies have been less conclusive (Spoont 1992).

Studies using functional imaging (i.e., PET scans) have also shown decreased cerebral glucose metabolism in the frontal lobes to be associated with aggressive behavior. One study of psychiatric patients with violent histories showed that all of the patients studied had decreased blood flow to the left temporal lobes and that two of the four patients also had decreased blood flow to the frontal lobes (Volkow and Tancredi 1987). A larger study showed that of the population studied, 22 homicide offenders had bilaterally decreased glucose metabolism in both the superior and anterior medial frontal cortex (corresponding to Brodmann areas 32 and 12) and a trend toward decreased metabolism in the orbital frontal cortex compared with normal controls (Raine et al. 1994). Two other studies using PET scanning have shown decreased glucose metabolism in the orbital frontal cortex (Brodmann area 11) as well as in areas nearby such as the middle frontal or inferior frontal cortex (Goyer et al. 1994a).

Overall, many of the PET scan data to date appear to support the hypothesis that decreased control of impulsivity and aggression seems to correlate with decreased metabolic activity in the orbital frontal cortex, with some additional decrease in the surrounding cortical areas and in the temporal lobes. For example, in a PET study of 17 patients with personality disorders and 43 normal controls engaged in an auditory CPT, Goyer and colleagues (1994a, 1994b) found decreased rates of glucose metabolism in BPD patients compared with controls in the frontal cortex in a plane 81 mm above the canthomeatal line (CML) and increased rates in a plane 55 mm above the CML. They also reported a correlation between the degree of metabolic activity in the anterior medial frontal and left anterior frontal regions of this lower plane and life history of aggression in patients with personality disorders. To determine whether BPD was a variant of temporal lobe epilepsy, de la Fuente et al. (1994) used PET to compare 10 borderline patients with 15 age-matched controls, looking for the temporal lobe asymmetry in metabolic activity that is characteristic of temporal lobe epilepsy. They found no support for the epilepsy hypothesis but instead found a trend for an increased rate of glucose metabolism in the posterior region of the right temporal lobe in BPD patients. Although not explicitly studying patients with antisocial personality disorder, Raine (1994) used PET to study a group of murderers pleading not guilty by reason of insanity. The subjects performed a standardized CPT during isotope uptake. The investigators found lower rates of glucose metabolism in the lateral and medial prefrontal cortex in murderers compared with controls. Overall, many of the PET scan data to date appear to support the hypothesis that decreased control of impulsivity and aggression seems to correlate with decreased metabolic activity in the orbital frontal cortex, with some additional decrease in the surrounding cortical areas and in the temporal lobes.

As has been shown, both reduced serotonin activity and decreased metabolic activity in the orbital frontal cortex appear to correlate with increased impulsivity and aggression. The next question to investigate, then, is whether there are abnormalities in the serotonin activity in the areas that show decreased metabolic activity. It has been shown that the frontal cortex, as well as the temporal lobe and the amygdala, are widely innervated by serotonergic neurons that project from the raphe nucleus in the medulla. In addition, the prefrontal cortex has been found to have high concentrations of 5-HT_2 and 5-HT_{1a} receptors and transporter sites. Other evidence of the relationship between serotonergic activity and the areas of interest are the observations that in patients with frontotemporal contusions, the concentrations of 5-hydroxyindoleacetic acid (5-HIAA) are significantly lower than in patients with more diffuse contusions (Van Woerken et al. 1977). Finally, PET studies done recently show that fenfluramine, when given to normal controls, can increase metabolism in their frontal and temporal lobes, especially in the orbital frontal cortex (Mann et al. 1996). These studies evidence the extent of serotonergic activity in those areas.

Animal and human studies have shown regional differences in serotonin activity to be correlated with impulsivity and aggression (Arango and Mann 1992), as well as suicidal behavior and depression. One study in particular has shown that the number of 5-HT_2 receptors in the posterior orbitofrontal cortex, medial frontal cortex, and amygdala were related inversely to aggressive behavior in monkeys (Raleigh and Brammer 1993). One recent study by Mann et al. (1996) showed decreased metabolic responsivity to a fenfluramine challenge in the prefrontal cortices of moderately depressed patients in comparison with normal controls. (Normal controls showed increases in glucose metabolism in the left prefrontal cortex and temporoparietal cortex and decreases in the right prefrontal cortex; depressed patients did not demonstrate either significant increases or decreases in any area.) Their sample of depressed patients included patients with a history of personality disorders, as well as patients with a history of suicide attempts. However, given the small number of subjects in the study, the effect of these variables on the significance of the study cannot be determined.

Although substantial data show that aggression and impulsivity are associated with both decreased metabolism in the orbitofrontal cortex and abnormal serotonergic function, there is currently little direct evidence that these traits are due to abnormalities of serotonergic activity in the proposed areas. A pilot study at our center has attempted to ascertain such direct evidence. This study examined the difference in the metabolic response to a fenfluramine challenge using PET scan imaging in patients with a history of aggression and/or impulsivity as compared with normal controls. Six patients with impulsivity and/or aggression were compared with five normal volunteers. All subjects underwent a baseline PET scan initially. On a separate day, the subjects were given a challenge dose of fenfluramine and then subsequently underwent a second PET scan. The post-fenfluramine scans were compared with the baseline scans, and no significant differences were seen in the baseline glucose metabolism between the normal controls and the patients. The controls showed increased metabolism in the orbital frontal and adjacent ventral medial frontal cortex, cingulate, and inferior parietal cortex after fenfluramine administration compared with baseline. In contrast, the impulsive aggressive patients appeared to have significantly blunted responses to fenfluramine in glucose metabolism in the orbital frontal, adjacent ventral, and cingulate cortex, but not in the inferior parietal cortex, when compared with normal subjects.

Hence the combination of a serotonergic challenge with PET scan imaging holds promise for helping to delineate some of the biological abnormalities underlying the symptoms of impulsivity and poor control of aggression as seen in a subset of the personality disorders. Other combinations of drug challenges or cognitive testing in conjunction with functional imaging could also potentially lead to a greater understanding of the different aspects and traits involved in the diagnoses of the personality disorders.

Cognitive Science Strategies

The study of cognitive processes including executive function, learning, abstraction, language, and attention has been revolutionized over the last two decades. A better understanding of these cognitive processes has also made possible an appreciation of individual differences in cognitive processing that may play a role in differences in personality style. When extreme, these differences may indeed constitute the basis for a personality disorder. For example, a relative impairment in working memory may make it difficult for an individual to hold "on-line" representations of others in their environment, impairing their capacity for interpersonal interactions. Attentional problems may make it difficult for them to engage interpersonally in a sustained fashion. For example, one schizotypal patient noted that "very soon after I start a conversation I notice people are no longer with me, probably because my mind has gone elsewhere and they can tell that I'm no longer able to pay attention to them." People who are unable to read the nonverbal and verbal cues that are a necessary ingredient of interpersonal interactions quickly find themselves feeling out of place. Cognitive distortions not only interfere with successful interpersonal relations but when more severe can also result in distorted cognitions or perceptions about the world. These views may take the form of unusual beliefs, referential ideas, or perceptual distortions.

The new tools of cognitive neuroscience have enabled investigators to critically investigate these cognitive processes in patients with personality disorders and link these processes to specific personality traits. Thus a new way to approach the biological basis of these disorders is to investigate the neurochemistry and pharmacology of cognition and cognitive impairment in these patients, and we can begin with patients with SPD. This method has implications for the study of not only personality disorders but also schizophrenia.

Studies to Date

The odd cluster personality disorders are characterized by people with a pervasive interpersonal isolation. Patients in this cluster are perceived by others as eccentric and loners. Paranoid and schizoid personality disorders have been little investigated, but much research has been carried out into SPD, the third and most severe personality disorder in this category. It is evident that abnormalities in cognitive functioning may relate to personality style, and cognitive impairment may be seen as central to the pathology of these eccentric personality disorders. Cognitive organization may be described as the ability to organize information and apply it appropriately in order to interact with the environment in a reasonable way. Difficulties in this realm of cognition are manifested in both the psychotic-like symptoms of SPD and the less dramatic impairment in interpersonal interaction that characterizes this disorder. Cognitive organization is most profoundly impaired in chronic schizophrenia, where reality testing is severely distorted. It now appears that negative symptoms and cognitive impairment may be more relevant in the production of functional disability than are positive or psychotic-like symptoms (Green 1996). Patients with SPD are generally free from factors that confound the study of schizophrenic patients, such as chronic psychosis, institutionalization, and effects of neuroleptic medication, and these patients have already proven quite amenable to pharmacological challenge studies. Because they share the cognitive dysfunction of the schizophrenic spectrum but have less severe and apparently more readily reversible dysfunction, they represent the ideal group to which to apply the principles of cognitive neuropsychology. The dramatic cluster personality disorders may also be viewed in terms of cognitive impairment in that patients, particularly borderline subjects, show abnormalities on neuropsychological testing; these abnormalities may be responsible for symptoms such as confusion, distortions, forgetfulness, odd reasoning, and failure to learn and change. Further, the distractibility and poor concentration of patients with other disorders, such as attention-deficit disorder, who clinically show some similarities with dramatic cluster personality disorders may also have some similarity with regard to the neurochemical basis.

Cognitive Impairment in SPD

Cognitive impairment has been clearly documented in both SPD and schizophrenia (Gold and Harvey 1993) and has been associated with deficit symptoms. The impairment includes abnormalities of executive function, visuospatial working memory, verbal memory, and sustained attention.

Performance is impaired on tests of frontal lobe function such as the Wisconsin Card Sorting Test (WCST) (Heaton 1985), a test of ability to shift set, and on the Trails B test (Lezak 1983) in patients with SPD (Trestman et al. 1995) and in those with schizophrenia. Wechsler Adult Intelligence Scale—Revised (WAIS-R) (Wechsler 1981) vocabulary and block design performance are not impaired among these patients, however, and this finding decreases the likelihood of a global impairment in functioning.

The involvement of dopamine receptors in cognition, specifically in the mnemonic processes of the prefrontal cortex, is supported by the observation that dopamine antagonists administered in the frontal cortex in primates results in impaired working memory as measured by a delayed-response task (Sawaguchi and Goldman-Rakic 1991). Deficits in working memory form a critical part of the cognitive deficit in schizophrenia. SPD patients have also shown deficits on a visuospatial working memory task (Lees-Roitman et al. 1996), as well as reductions in verbal memory (Voglmaier et al. 1996). Patients with schizophrenia show deficits in learning and memory (Saykin et al. 1991), and their relatives exhibit impairments in verbal learning, recall, and recognition (Lyons et al. 1995). These findings suggest that the biological basis of cognitive dysfunction in schizophrenic patients may also be present in their relatives but in an attenuated form, a form similar to the less severely affected patients with SPD.

Much work has been carried out on the attention system of the human brain, the importance of attention being its function in connecting the description of processes used in cognitive science with the anatomic level employed in neuroscience (Posner 1990). It has been proposed that attentional impairment is a core deficit in schizophrenia. The CPT, a test of sustained attention, is abnormal in patients with schizophrenia, patients with SPD (Harvey et al. 1996), and volunteers with schizotypal traits. Abnormalities on this test are correlated with social isolation in children of schizophrenic patients (Cornblatt et al. 1992). Further, in patients at risk for schizophrenia, abnormalities on the CPT in childhood have been shown to be related to schizotypal traits in adulthood (Cornblatt et al. 1992), and this finding provides support for the hypothesis that poor attention and negative symptoms are associated. The Backward Masking Test (Lezak 1983) also examines information processing and has, in some studies, been found to be abnormal in schizophrenic and schizotypal patients, although not in one recent study of schizotypal patients (Harvey et al. 1996).

Event-related potentials, which provide a further measure of selective attention, are abnormal in schizophrenia; this abnormality has been associated with negative symptoms. Patients with SPD also exhibit abnormalities in event-related potentials, and in one recent study patients with SPD showed significant abnormalities in p300 topography over the left posterior temporal area (Salisbury et al. 1996). The abnormality in SPD is less marked than that in schizophrenia (Trestman et al. 1996), is not specific to SPD, and is found in other patients such as those with BPD (Kutcher et al. 1989).

More than half of schizophrenic patients evidence abnormal eye tracking, compared with less than 10% of the normal population. Abnormal eye movements are seen in the relatives of schizophrenic patients (Holzman et al. 1984) and in patients with SPD. Furthermore, in schizotypal patients (Siever et al. 1990), as well as volunteers, abnormal eye movements are associated with deficit symptoms (Siever et al. 1994).

Autonomic responses to environmental stimuli are measured by the orienting response. This response is abnormal in schizophrenia and SPD, in that these patients show hypoarousal to stimuli. Visual reaction time also tests information processing and is abnormal in schizophrenic patients and patients with SPD; both groups show crossover, which represents attentional impairment (Siever 1985).

The brains of schizophrenic patients show structural abnormalities including increased ventricle size, increased ventricular brain ratios, and cortical atrophy. SPD patients also show increased ventricular size, and in one study this increased ventricular size was associated with deficit symptoms (Siever et al. 1993). Structural abnormalities have been correlated with decreased plasma homovanillic acid (HVA) levels and impaired performance on neuropsychological tasks (Siever et al. 1993).

Cognitive Impairment in BPD

Neurocognitive abnormalities have been noted in patients with dramatic cluster personality disorders. These abnormalities include poor performance on the Trails B test, the WAIS digit symbol test (Wechsler 1981) and the Benton figure drawing test (Lezak 1983), among others. These tests are sensitive to brain dysfunction but are not specific for any one brain area (Burgess and Zarconi 1992). Neuropsychological testing also reveals BPD patients to perform poorly during the process of visual discrimination and filtering and to have difficulty recalling complex material. Both of these tests may be sensitive to abnormalities in the dominant temporal lobe (O'Leary et al. 1991). The performance of BPD patients has been found to be significantly impaired on visuospatial tasks, and this impairment does not appear to be related to depression, psychomotor, or attentional problems (Judd and Ruff 1993). These findings have important clinical implications; the BPD patient may be unable to learn and integrate information meaningfully and thus be unable to retrieve it. These difficulties may lead to poor capacity for representation. Finally, it has been suggested that subtle organic factors may exist in some of these patients. Significantly lower IQ scores have been found in these subjects in comparison with normal subjects; they also have significant impairment on visuomotor integration and figural memory (Swirsky-Sacchetti et al. 1993).

Implications

Strategies to Improve Cognition in SPD

In SPD, abnormalities on the WCST have been correlated with both deficit-type symptoms and decreased concentrations of plasma HVA. In relatives of schizophrenic patients with schizotypal traits, deficit symptoms have been significantly correlated with hypodopaminergia (Amin et al. 1997). Therefore, dopamine enhancement might reasonably be expected to improve cognitive impairment in SPD patients. The use of amphetamine, a dopamine agonist, represents a new strategy in the investigation of cognition in patients with personality disorders. Amphetamine was first noticed in 1938 to result in psychosis in some patients taking it for the treatment of narcolepsy. Later it was used as a research probe in schizophrenia, with varying results. The differential effects of amphetamine on positive and negative symptoms in schizophrenia were examined; results were confused by the fact that patients were being treated with neuroleptics (Cesarec and Nyman 1985). In the meantime the dopamine hypothesis of schizophrenia was updated to reflect the possibility that the psychotic symptoms of schizophrenia may be due to hyperdopaminergia and the negative symptoms the result of hypodopaminergia in the frontal cortex. If deficit-like symptoms (and cognitive impairment) in the schizophrenia spectrum are due to hypodopaminergia, then amphetamine should improve them. Administration of amphetamine to schizophrenic patients resulting in improvement on the WCST further implies that impaired executive function and hypofrontality are associated with hypodopaminergia (Daniel et al. 1991). In preliminary studies in a group of SPD patients, administration of amphetamine resulted in improved cognitive performance. In nine patients with SPD given 30 mg of amphetamine or placebo, seven improved on the WCST rate of perseverative errors with amphetamine (Siegel et al. 1996). One would expect that psychotic-like symptoms might worsen; however, more recent work shows that SPD patients selected solely on the basis of meeting SPD criteria do not show an increase in psychotic-like symptoms with amphetamine. This finding supports the hypothesis that patients with SPD may be less vulnerable to psychosis based on hyperdopaminergia due to protective factors such as perhaps reduced dopaminergic lability (L. J. Siever, unpublished data, April 1997).

Other strategies that may prove useful in clarifying and improving the cognitive deficits associated with personality disorder include the use of a selective D_1 agonist when it becomes available. Cumulatively, these data suggest that the study of cognition may provide important tools with which to characterize personality disorder traits, particularly those of the odd cluster.

Candidate Gene Strategies

Background

Traditionally, psychiatric genetics has been based primarily on strategies of linkage analyses for major Axis I disorders such as schizophrenia and bipolar disorder. However, new candidate gene strategies are gaining increasing favor in the exploration of psychiatric disorders and may be ideally suited to the investigation of the Axis II disorders. Candidate genes have already been fruitfully investigated in normal populations in relation to personality traits such as novelty seeking, neuroticism, and impulsivity. Candidate gene approaches have the power to detect relatively modest genetic contributions to phenotypic traits that may be better suited for personality traits that are likely to have multifactorial etiologies, including the interaction of a number of genes and the interaction of genes and environmental influences. The psychological traits themselves may be expressed in varying degrees of severity. If so, this factor would make classification of phenotypes as present or absent as with linkage studies somewhat more problematic. For candidate gene studies, subjects with a specific genotype reflecting the presence of a particular allele can be compared with regard to their value on a quantitative trait dimension with those with a complementary allele. Furthermore, it becomes possible to evaluate variability in severity of this trait that accompanies the homozygote and the heterozygote for the particular allele. The candidate gene approach also allows for building on empirical research identifying neurobiological mechanisms in the pathogenesis of a particular personality disorder dimension, such as impulsivity, where the serotonergic system is implicated. In the case of serotonergic-related genes, alleles for the serotonin transporter, the synthetic enzyme tryptophan hydroxylase, and a variety of serotonergic receptors have been identified. Studies to date make it appear likely that up to 10 or more genes may account for the genetic heritability of personality disorder traits such as anxiety-related personality traits or impulsivity. Thus, candidate gene approaches may be extraordinarily useful for detecting modest genetic effects in known neurobiological systems related to personality dimensions such as impulsivity, affective reactivity, or anxiety or inhibition. Candidate gene association studies can be strengthened by the analyses of siblings or even parents, which allow stronger inferences to be made about the association of the candidate gene of interest on the particular behavior.

Impulsive aggression is an especially appropriate behavior in which to use the candidate gene approach, because strong evidence has implicated the serotonin system in the control of impulsive aggressive behavior. Serotonergic abnormalities have been observed in personality disorder patients and depressed patients, volunteers, and violent alcoholic offenders, as demonstrated by a range of indexes from metabolite studies of cerebrospinal fluid (CSF) 5-HIAA to challenge with serotonergic-enhancing agents such as fenfluramine (Linnoila et al. 1994; O'Keane et al. 1992; Siever et al. 1993). This issue is discussed in more detail in Chapter 1 of this text. These observations make it possible to narrow the selection of appropriate candidate genes to those involved in serotonergic activity, which can be considered a promising tool to test for associations with impulsive aggression.

A further theoretical consideration underlying the candidate gene approach in impulsive aggression comes from evidence that impulsive aggression is at least partially heritable. Preliminary data from monozygotic-dizygotic twin studies and family studies suggest that the traits of impulsive or assertive aggression are significantly heritable (Coccaro et al. 1993, 1994; Torgersen 1992). In light of the heritability of impulsive aggression, in addition to the association of defects in serotonin functioning associated with this behavior, a much more compelling case can be made for the investigation of genetic differences in determinants of serotonergic function—such as synthesis, metabolism, and receptor sensitivity—that may contribute to different susceptibilities to impulsive aggression.

Studies to Date

Numerous polymorphisms related to gene products involved in serotonin synthesis, reuptake, metabolism, and receptors have been identified in nonhuman primates (Raleigh et al. 1994) and human subjects. The serotonin-related gene best studied for its relationship to impulsive aggressive behavior is the gene coding for tryptophan hydroxylase (TPH), the first enzyme involved in the synthesis of serotonin. A polymorphism in the gene on chromosome 11 coding for TPH has been identified, and the two alleles have been designated L and U, with frequencies of 0.40 and 0.60, respectively, in unrelated Caucasians. In a Finnish cohort of violent alcohol offenders, the L TPH allele was associated with reduced CSF 5-HIAA concentrations and a history of suicide attempts (Nielsen et al. 1994, 1995). Evidence from our group (New et al., in press) suggests that in male Caucasian patients with personality disorders, the LL genotype was associated with significantly higher total scores on the Buss-Durkee Hostility Inventory (BDHI) (Buss et al. 1956) (45.3 ± 9.8) compared with Caucasian males with the UL or UU genotype (32.9 ± 13.5; $t = 2.38$, df $= 19$, $P < .03$), although this association was not found in women. No significant association was found between the LL genotype and a history of suicide attempt or impulsive BPD traits in this sample. It should be noted, however, that the functional significance of this polymorphism has yet to be proven. Because this is an intronic polymorphism (intronic areas of a gene are not directly involved in coding for a protein), the two alleles do not code for a different protein. Another gene that has been implicated in the susceptibility to impulsive aggression is the gene coding for the serotonin transporter, *SLC6A4*. The serotonin transporter is important in serotonergic functioning in that it plays a central role in the termination of serotonin neurotransmission and represents a site of antidepressant activity. Furthermore, twin studies suggest that platelet serotonin uptake, mediated by an identical serotonin transporter receptor to that found in the brain, may be partially genetically controlled (Meltzer and Arora 1986). One polymorphism in the promoter region of the serotonin transporter gene has been demonstrated to have functional significance in coding for either high- or low-level transporter production. This polymorphism was recently found to be associated with a high degree of harm avoidance in a racially mixed sample (Lesch et al. 1996). To replicate this finding, we combined racial and gender groups and obtained genotype data on 74 patients; 21 patients had l/l (long, long) and 16 patients had s/s (short, short) polymorphisms. In our preliminary data, patients who were homozygous for the short allele had significantly higher harm avoidance scores compared with patients who were homozygous for the long allele. Patients who were heterozygous were intermediate (New et al., in press).

Additionally, an intronic polymorphism (a polymorphism in a region not translated into protein) in the serotonin transporter gene *(SLC6A4)* has been identified (Lesch et al. 1994). Frequent variants of this allele have either 10 or 12 copies of a 17-base repeat. The 10-copy allele had a frequency of 0.47 in a general population in Germany. Our preliminary data suggest that the 10-copy allele may be associated with increased measures of impulsivity in patients with personality disorders (New et al., in press).

Implications

The approach of identifying the relationship between serotonin-related genotypes and impulsive aggressive behavior is promising because it may elucidate the mechanism underlying the susceptibility to impulsive aggression. Although abnormalities in serotonin-related genes have been associated with impulsive aggressive behavior, the identification of behavioral differences by genotype in a specific receptor subtype may help to clarify specific pathophysiology. Furthermore, it may be possible in the future to identify by genotype individuals at risk for aggressive behavior and thereby target treatment strategies to a high-risk population. The candidate gene approach would also be used to explore the relationships between other neurotransmitter systems such as the dopamine system and psychotic-like symptoms.

Conclusions

Although most of the biological strategies described in this chapter have only recently been applied to the personality disorders, the results of these studies are promising in suggesting that the new techniques of neuroimaging, genetics, and cognitive science may enhance our understanding of core dimensions of the personality disorders. These techniques may permit a more focused study of the brain systems implicated in cognitive disorganization, dyscontrol of aggression, affective instability, and anxiety. Utilization of these techniques may change and broaden our understanding of the genetic and psychosocial antecedents of these personality dysfunctions.

It is increasingly understood that the pathogenesis of the personality disorders is multifactorial in etiology and is probably based on the interaction of multiple genes with environmental antecedents such as abuse or trauma in the extreme cases. This issue is further elaborated on in Chapter 5 of this text. Ultimately, the application of these techniques in conjunction with longitudinal studies may enable us to better understand the mechanisms of maladaptive personality development, which in turn may eventually lead to improvement in our capacity to intervene effectively both psychopharmacologically and psychotherapeutically.

References

Akiskal HS: Subaffective disorders: dysthymic, cyclothymic, and bipolar II disorders in the "borderline" realm. Psychiatr Clin North Am 4:25–46, 1981

Amin F, Coccaro EF, Mitropoulou V, et al: Plasma HVA in schizotypal personality disorder, in Plasma Homovanillic Acid Studies in Schizophrenia: Implications for Presynaptic Dopamine Dysfunction. Edited by Friedhoff AJ, Amin F. Washington, DC, American Psychiatric Press, 1997, pp 133–149

Arango V, Mann J: Relevance of serotonergic postmortem studies to suicidal behavior. International Review of Psychiatry 4:131–140, 1992

Azmitia EC, Liao B, Chen YS: Increase of tryptophan hydroxylase enzyme protein by dexamethasone in adrenalectomized rat midbrain. J Neurosci 13:5041–5055, 1993

Bandettini PA, Wong EC, Binder JR, et al: Functional MRI imaging using the BOLD approach: dynamic characteristics and data analysis methods, in Diffusion and Perfusion Magnetic Resonance Imaging. Edited by Le Bihan D. New York, Raven, 1995, pp 335–349

Buchsbaum MS, Wu J, Siegel BV, et al: Effect of sertraline on regional metabolic rate in patients with affective disorder. Biol Psychiatry 41:15–22, 1997

Burgess JW, Zarconi VP: Cognitive impairment in dramatic personality disorders (letter). Am J Psychiatry 149:136, 1992

Buss AH, Durkee A, Baer MB: The measurement of hostility in clinical situations. J Abnorm Psychol 52:84–86, 1956

Cesarec Z, Nyman AK: Differential response to amphetamine in schizophrenia. Acta Psychiatr Scand 71:523–538, 1985

Coccaro EF, Bergman CS, McLean GE: Heritability of irritable impulsiveness: a study of twins reared together and apart. Psychiatry Res 48:229–242, 1993

Coccaro E, Silverman J, Klar H, et al: Familial correlates of reduced central serotonergic system function in patients with personality disorders. Arch Gen Psychiatry 51:318–324, 1994

Cornblatt BA, Lenzenweger MF, Dworkin RH, et al: Childhood attentional dysfunctions predict social deficits in unaffected adults at risk for schizophrenia. Br J Psychiatry 161(suppl 18):59–64, 1992

Damasio H, Grabowski T, Frank R, et al: The return of Phineas Gage: clues about the brain from the skull of a famous patient. Science 264:1102–1105, 1994

Daniel DG, Weinberger DR, Jones DW, et al: The effect of amphetamine on regional cerebral blood flow during cognitive activation in schizophrenia. J Neurosci 11:1907–1917, 1991 de la Fuente JM, Lotstra F, Goldman S, et al: Temporal glucose metabolism in borderline personality disorder. Psychiatry Res 55:237–245, 1994

George MS, Ketter TA, Parekh PI, et al: Brain activity during transient sadness and happiness in healthy women. Am J Psychiatry 152:341–351, 1995

Gold JM, Harvey PD: Cognitive deficits in schizophrenia. Psychiatr Clin North Am 16:295–312, 1993

Goyer PF, Andreason PJ, Semple WE, et al: Positron-emission tomography and personality disorders. Neuropsychopharmacology 10:21–28, 1994a

Goyer PF, Konicki PE, Schulz SC: Brain imaging in personality disorders, in Biological and Neurobehavioral Studies of Borderline Personality Disorder. Edited by Silk KR. Washington, DC, American Psychiatric Press, 1994b, pp 109–126

Green MF: What are the functional consequences of neurocognitive deficits in schizophrenia? Am J Psychiatry 153:321–330, 1996

Grossman R, Yehuda R, Siever LJ: Trauma and HPA axis activity in personality disorders and normal controls. Paper presented at the annual meeting of the American Psychiatric Association (abstract NR551), San Diego, CA, May 1997

Gunderson JG, Sabo AN: The phenomenological and conceptual interface between borderline personality disorder and PTSD. Am J Psychiatry 150:19–27, 1993

Hamilton M: A rating scale for depression. J Neurol Neurosurg Psychiatry 23:56–62, 1960

Harvey PD, Keefe RS, Mitroupoulou V, et al: Information-processing markers of vulnerability to schizophrenia: performance of patients with schizotypal and nonschizotypal personality disorders. Psychiatry Res 60:49–56, 1996

Heaton R: Wisconsin Card Sorting Test. Odessa, TX, Psychological Assessments Resources, 1985

Heinrichs W: Frontal cerebral lesions and violent incidents in chronic neuropsychiatric patients. Biol Psychiatry 25:174–178, 1989

Herman J: Trauma and Recovery. New York, Basic Books, 1992

Herman JL, Perry JC, van der Kolk BA: Childhood trauma in borderline personality disorder. Am J Psychiatry 146:490–495, 1989

Holcomb HH, Links J, Smith C, et al: Positron emission tomography: measuring the metabolic and neurochemical characteristics of the living human nervous system, in Brain Imaging: Applications in Psychiatry. Edited by Andreasen NC. Washington, DC, American Psychiatric Press, 1989, pp 235–270

Holzman PS, Solomon CM, Levin S, et al: Pursuit eye movement dysfunctions in schizophrenia. Arch Gen Psychiatry 41:136–139, 1984

Intrator J, Hare R, Stritzke P, et al: A brain imaging (single photon emission computerized tomography) study of semantic and affective processing in psychopaths. Biol Psychiatry 42:96–103, 1997

Irwin W, Davidson RJ, Lowe MJ, et al: Human amygdala activation detected with echo-planar functional magnetic resonance imaging. Neuroreport 7:1765–1769, 1996

Judd PH, Ruff RM: Neuropsychological dysfunction in borderline personality disorder. Journal of Personality Disorders 7:275–284, 1993

Kutcher SP, Blackwood DH, Gaskell DF, et al: Auditory p300 does not differentiate borderline personality disorder from schizotypal personality disorder. Biol Psychiatry 26:766–774, 1989

Laaris N, Haj-Dahmane S, Hamon M, et al: Glucocorticoid receptor–mediated inhibition by corticosterone of 5-HT$_{1A}$ autoreceptor functioning in the rat dorsal raphe nucleus. Neuropharmacology 34:1201–1210, 1995

Lee CC, Jack CR, Riederer SJ: Use of functional magnetic resonance imaging. Neurosurg Clin N Am 7:665–683, 1996

Lees-Roitman SE, Keefe RSE, Dupre RL, et al: Visuospatial working memory in schizotypal personality disorder (abstract). Biol Psychiatry 39:577, 1996

Lesch K, Balling U, Gross J, et al: Organization of the human serotonin transporter gene. J Neurol Transm Genet 95:157–162, 1994

Lesch K, Bengel D, Heils A, et al: Association of anxiety-related traits with a polymorphism in the serotonin transporter gene regulatory region. Science 274:1527–1531, 1996

Lezak MD: Neuropsychological Assessment, 2nd Edition. Edited by Toglia MP, Battig WF. New York, Oxford University Press, 1983

Linnoila M, Virkkunen M, George T, et al: Serotonin, behavior, and alcohol, in Toward a Molecular Basis of Alcohol Use and Abuse. Edited by Jansson B, Jornvall H, Rydberg U, et al. Basel, Switzerland, Birkhauser Verlag, 1994, pp 154–163

Lyons MJ, Toomey R, Seidman LJ, et al: Verbal learning and memory in relatives of schizophrenics: preliminary findings. Biol Psychiatry 37:750–753, 1995

Mann JJ, Malone KM, Diehl DJ, et al: Demonstration in vivo of reduced serotonin responsivity in the brain of untreated depressed patients. Am J Psychiatry 153:174–182, 1996

Meaney MJ, Aitken DH, Sharma S, et al: Post-natal handling increases hippocampal type II, glucocorticoid receptors and enhances adreno-cortical negative-feedback efficacy in the rat. Neuroendocrinology 50:597–604, 1989

Meijer OC, de Kloet RE: A role for the mineralocorticoid receptor in a rapid and transient suppression of hippocampal 5-HT$_{1A}$ receptor mRNA by corticosterone. Eur J Pharmacol 266:255–261, 1994

Meltzer H, Arora R: Platelet markers of suicidality. Ann N Y Acad Sci 487:271–280, 1986

Mitchell JB, Rowe W, Boksa P, et al: Serotonin regulates type II corticosteroid receptor binding in hippocampal cell cultures. J Neurosci 10:1745–1752, 1990

New AS, Yehuda R, Steinberg B, et al: Self-reported abuse and biological measures in personality disorders (abstract). Biol Psychiatry 39:535, 1996

New AS, Gelernter J, Yovell Y, et al: Tryptophan hydroxylase genotype is associated with impulsive aggression measures: a preliminary study. Neuropsychiatric Genetics (in press)

Nielsen DA, Goldman D, Virkkunen M, et al: Suicidality and 5-hydroxyindoleacetic acid concentration associated with a tryptophan hydroxylase polymorphism. Arch Gen Psychiatry 51:34–38, 1994

Nielsen D, Stefanisko K, Virkkunen M, et al: Association of tryptophan hydroxylase genotype with suicidal behavior in Finns: a replication study. Paper presented at the 34th Annual Meeting of the American College of Neuropsychopharmacology, San Juan, Puerto Rico, December 1995

Novotny S, Lowry MT: Short-term and long-term effects of p-chloroamphetamine on hippocampal serotonin and corticosteroid receptor levels. Brain Res 684:19–25, 1995

O'Keane V, Moloney E, O'Neill H, et al: Blunted prolactin responses to d-fenfluramine in sociopathy: evidence for subsensitivity of central serotonergic function. Br J Psychiatry 160:643–646, 1992

O'Leary KM, Brouwers P, Gardner DL, et al: Neuropsychological testing of patients with borderline personality disorder. Am J Psychiatry 148:106–111, 1991

Paris J, Zweig-Frank H: A critical review of the role of childhood sexual abuse in the etiology of borderline personality disorder. Can J Psychiatry 37:125–128, 1992

Posner MI: The attention system of the human brain. Annu Rev Neurosci 13:25–42, 1990

Raine A, Sheard C, Reynolds GP, et al: Pre-frontal structural and functional deficits associated with individual differences in schizotypal personality. Schizophr Res 7:237–247, 1992

Raine A, Buchsbaum M, Stanley J, et al: Selective reductions in prefrontal glucose metabolism in murderers. Biol Psychiatry 36:365–373, 1994

Raleigh MJ, Brammer GL: Individual differences in serotonin-2 receptors and social behavior in monkeys (abstract). Society for Neuroscience 19:592, 1993

Raleigh MJ, Nielsen DA, McGuire MT, et al: Behavioral and biochemical correlates of genotypic differences in Vervet monkeys. Proceedings of the American College of Neuropsychopharmacology, San Juan, Puerto Rico, December 1994

Salisbury DF, Voglmaier MM, Seidman LJ, et al: Topographic abnormalities of P3 in schizotypal personality disorder. Biol Psychiatry 40:165–172, 1996

Sawaguchi T, Goldman-Rakic P: D_1 dopamine receptors in prefrontal cortex: involvement in working memory. Science 251:947–950, 1991

Saykin AJ, Gur RC, Gur RE, et al: Neuropsychological function in schizophrenia. Arch Gen Psychiatry 48:618–624, 1991

Schwartz JM, Stoessel PW, Baxter LR, et al: Systematic changes in cerebral glucose metabolic rate after successful treatment of obsessive-compulsive disorder. Arch Gen Psychiatry 53:109–113, 1996

Siegel BV, Trestman RL, O'Flaithbheartaigh S, et al: D-amphetamine challenge effects on Wisconsin Card Sort Test: performance in schizotypal personality disorder. Schizophr Res 20:29–32, 1996

Siever LJ: Biological markers in schizotypal personality disorder. Schizophr Bull 11:564–575, 1985

Siever LJ: The biology of the boundaries of schizophrenia, in Advances in Neuropsychiatry and Psychopharmacology, Vol 1: Schizophrenia Research. Edited by Tamminga CA, Schulz CS. New York, Raven, 1991, pp 181–191

Siever LJ, Keefe R, Bernstein DP, et al: Eye tracking impairment in clinically identified patients with schizotypal personality disorder. Am J Psychiatry 147:740–745, 1990

Siever LJ, Kalus OF, Keefe RS: The boundaries of schizophrenia. Psychiatr Clin North Am 16:217–244, 1993

Siever LJ, Friedman L, Moskowitz J, et al: Eye movement impairment and schizotypal pathology. Am J Psychiatry 151:1209–1215, 1994

Soares JC, Mann JJ: The anatomy of mood disorders: review of structural neuroimaging studies. Biol Psychiatry 41:86–106, 1997

Spoont MR: Modulatory role of serotonin in the neural information processing: implications for human psychopathology. Psychol Bull 112:330–350, 1992

Swirsky-Sacchetti T, Gorton G, Samuel S, et al: Neuropsychological function in borderline personality disorder. J Clin Psychol 49:385–396, 1993

Torgersen S: Genetics in borderline conditions. Acta Psychiatr Scand Suppl 379:19–25, 1992

Trestman RL, Keefe RS, Mitropoulou V, et al: Cognitive function and biological correlates of cognitive performance in schizotypal personality disorder. Psychiatry Res 59:127–136, 1995

Trestman RL, Horvath T, Kalus O, et al: Event-related potentials in schizotypal personality disorder. J Neuropsychiatry Clin Neurosci 8:33–40, 1996

Van Woerken TCAM, Teelken AW, Minderhoud JM: Difference in neu-rotransmitter metabolism in frontotemporal-lobe contusion and dif-fuse cerebral contusion. Lancet 1:812–813, 1977

Voglmaier MM, Seidman LJ, Salisbury DF, et al: Learning and memory in schizotypal personality disorder. Paper presented at the annual meeting of the American Psychiatric Association, New York, May 1996

Volkow ND, Tancredi L: Neural substrates of violent behavior: a pre-liminary study with positron emission tomography. Br J Psychiatry 151:668–673, 1987

Wechsler D: Wechsler Adult Intelligence Scale—Revised. San Antonio, TX, Psychological Corporation, 1981

Weston S, Siever LJ: Biologic correlates of personality disorder. Journal of Personality Disorders 7(suppl):129–148, 1993

Yehuda R: Neuroendocrinology of trauma and PTSD, in Psychological Trauma. Edited by Yehuda R. Washington, DC, American Psychiatric Press, 1998

Zanarini MC, Gunderson JG, Marino MF, et al: Childhood experiences of borderline patients. Compr Psychiatry 30:18–25, 1989

Chapter 3

The Genetics and Psychobiology of the Seven-Factor Model of Personality

C. Robert Cloninger, M.D.

Understanding the psychobiology of personality has been a difficult challenge because the functional organization of brain systems is complex. Fortunately, the principles of genetic transmission are sufficiently simple that a unique model of the architecture of personality can be specified (Cloninger 1987, 1994a). I approached this problem through a series of steps reviewed in this chapter. First, I described a model of the genetic structure of personality based on twin and adoption studies of personality in humans and learning abilities in animals (Cloninger 1986, 1987). Second, I proposed a psychobiological model of learning abilities underlying human personality traits based on neuropharmacological studies of humans and animals from a phylogenetic perspective (Cloninger 1987, 1994a, 1995). Third, many independent investigators and I then evaluated the psychometric properties of quantitative tests for measuring personality and its disorders in the general population as well as in many clinical samples (Cloninger et al. 1994). This assessment produced evidence of the validity of two tests called the Tridimensional Personality Questionnaire (TPQ) (Cloninger 1987) and the more comprehensive Temperament and Character Inventory (TCI) (Cloninger et al. 1993) that was developed after

---

This work was supported in part by National Institutes of Health Grants MH31302, MH46276, MH46280, MH54723, and AA08403

---

the initial work on the TPQ. More recently, extensive work has been carried out by many investigators internationally to characterize the neuroanatomy, neuropsychology, neurochemistry, and neurogenetics of human personality using the TPQ and TCI. The initial three phases of research are briefly reviewed, and then the current state of our knowledge of the genetics and psychobiology of personality is described. A surprising amount of consistent information has emerged as the result of the availability of a reliable, comprehensive, multidimensional model of human personality.

Personality can be defined as the dynamic organization of the psychobiological systems that modulate adaptation to experience (Cloninger 1987). A long tradition in psychology distinguishes two major domains of personality—temperament and character. According to early psychologists, temperament referred to our congenital emotional predisposition, whereas character was what people made of themselves intentionally (see Kant 1798/1974). To carry out psychobiological research, it is useful to operationalize this distinction in terms of individual differences in neuroadaptive processes. Accordingly, temperament can be defined as the automatic associative responses to basic emotional stimuli that determine habits and skills, whereas character refers to the self-aware concepts that influence our voluntary intentions and attitudes (Cloninger et al. 1993).

Psychosocial researchers have usually defined temperament as those components of personality that are heritable, developmentally stable, emotion based, or uninfluenced by sociocultural learning (Goldsmith et al. 1987). Fortunately, these four alternative definitions are highly convergent; recent work shows that all dimensions of temperament, defined as individual differences in emotion-based habit patterns, are moderately heritable, stable from childhood through adulthood, and structurally consistent in different cultures and ethnic groups (Cloninger 1995). About 50% of the variance in temperament among individuals is heritable and stable from childhood through adulthood (see Table 3–1).

In contrast, character is weakly heritable but moderately influenced by sociocultural learning. It matures in a stepwise man-

Table 3–1. Difference in learning, brain systems, and etiology between temperament and character

Learning variable	Temperament	Character
Form of learning		
Level of awareness	Automatic	Intentional
Type of activity	Habits, skills	Goals, values
Learning principle	Associative conditioning	Conceptual insight
Brain systems	Limbic system striatum	Neocortex hippocampus
Etiologic components		
Genetic heritability	40%–60%	10%–15%
Shared sibling environment	0	30%–35%
Random environment	40%–60%	40%–60%

ner from infancy through late adulthood, and the timing and rate of transition between levels of maturity are nonlinear functions of antecedent temperament configurations and sociocultural education (Svrakic et al. 1996).

Temperament and Character

The distinction between temperament and character appears to correspond to the dissociation of the major brain systems for procedural versus propositional memory and learning, as depicted in Figure 3–1 and documented in studies summarized in later tables and text. In other words, temperament involves individual differences in habit learning (i.e., procedural learning), whereas character involves differences in higher cognitive processing, such as concepts about self and relations to others. The distinction between these two major neural systems for adaptation to experience has had a variety of labels, such as percept versus concept, emotion versus volition, instinct versus will, and habit versus cognition. According to this psychobiological perspective, character development can be operationalized in terms of abstract symbolic processes that are most highly developed in humans, such as self-directed behavior, empathic social cooper-

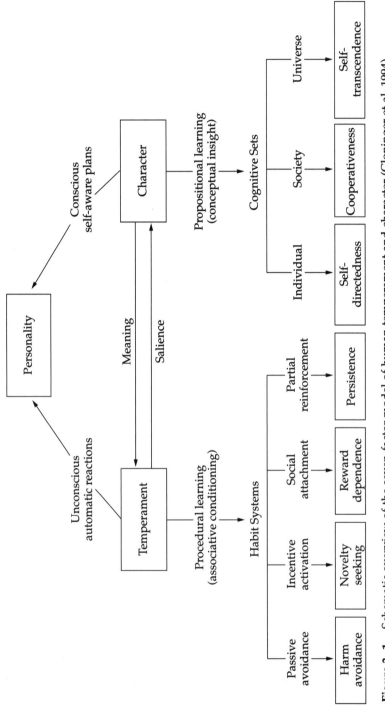

Figure 3–1. Schematic overview of the seven-factor model of human temperament and character (Cloninger et al. 1994).

ation, and creative symbolic invention. The hippocampal formation and cerebral neocortex are essential for encoding such concept-based, symbolic representations of experience. In contrast, temperament or basic emotionality can be operationalized in terms of associative habit learning that is perceptually based and well developed at an early age in nearly all vertebrates, even those without differentiation of the cerebral neocortex (Cloninger 1994b, 1995). Recent work described later shows that psychophysiological markers of neocortical processing, such as the P300 evoked potential to target stimuli, are correlated with individual differences in character but not temperament. This dissociation underscores the neurobiological importance of the distinction between temperament and character, which is neglected by factor analytically derived models of personality.

The four dimensions of human temperament correspond closely to those observed in other mammals, such as rodents and dogs (Wilsson and Sundgren 1997). Clinical descriptors of the four dimensions of human temperament and the three dimensions of character are summarized in Tables 3–2 and 3–3, respectively. Further details about factor structure, psychometrics, and relations to alternative models are provided in the TCI manual (Cloninger et al. 1994). In particular, the same multidimensional structure is observed in the general population (Cloninger et al. 1993) and in samples of psychiatric inpatients (Svrakic et al. 1993) or outpatients (Bayon et al. 1996).

The relationship of this multidimensional model to the clusters of DSM-IV (American Psychiatric Association 1994) personality disorders is shown in Table 3–4. All clusters of personality disorders are characterized by low scores in TCI self-directedness and cooperativeness. Deviations in temperament are associated with particular DSM-IV clusters: the anxious (C) cluster with high harm avoidance, the impulsive (B) cluster with high novelty seeking, and the aloof (A) cluster with low reward dependence. Furthermore, individual DSM-IV categories can be distinguished by a unique profile of TCI scores. For example, borderline personality disorder is characterized by an explosive temperament profile (i.e., high harm avoidance, high novelty

Table 3–2. Descriptors of individuals who score high and low on the four temperament dimensions

Temperament dimension	Descriptors of extreme variants	
	High	Low
Harm avoidance	Pessimistic	Optimistic
	Fearful	Daring
	Shy	Outgoing
	Fatigable	Energetic
Novelty seeking	Exploratory	Reserved
	Impulsive	Rigid
	Extravagant	Frugal
	Irritable	Stoic
Reward dependence	Sentimental	Critical
	Open	Aloof
	Warm	Detached
	Sympathetic	Independent
Persistence	Industrious	Lazy
	Determined	Spoiled
	Ambitious	Underachieving
	Perfectionistic	Pragmatic

Table 3–3. Descriptors of individuals who score high and low on the three character dimensions

Character dimension	Descriptors of extreme variants	
	High	Low
Self-directedness	Responsible	Blaming
	Purposeful	Aimless
	Resourceful	Inept
	Self-accepting	Vain
	Disciplined	Undisciplined
Cooperative	Tender hearted	Intolerant
	Empathic	Insensitive
	Helpful	Hostile
	Compassionate	Revengeful
	Principled	Opportunistic
Self-transcendent	Self-forgetful	Unimaginative
	Transpersonal	Controlling
	Spiritual	Materialistic
	Enlightened	Possessive
	Idealistic	Practical

Table 3–4. Correlations between Temperament and Character Inventory (TCI) scales and number of DSM-III-R personality disorder symptoms

TCI dimension	DSM-III-R personality disorder symptom counts by cluster			
	Total	Anxious	Impulsive	Aloof
Harm avoidant	+	+ +		+
Novelty seeking	+		+ +	
Reward dependent				− −
Persistent				
Self-directed	− − −	− −	− −	− −
Cooperative	− −	−	− −	− −
Self-transcendent				

Source. Goldman et al. 1994; Nagoshi et al. 1992; Svrakic et al. 1993.

seeking, and low reward dependence) together with low character scores. Such multidimensional decomposition allows a clinician to make mutually exclusive classifications without the usual problem of multiple overlapping diagnoses using ambiguous DSM-IV checklists.

Neurobiological Basis of the Structure of Procedural Learning

Neuropharmacological studies of animals, often rodents, and lesion and stimulation studies have provided explicit hypotheses for testing the relationships among stimulus-response learning and temperament. These hypotheses are summarized in Table 3–5 for all four temperament dimensions. This psychobiological learning model is based on neuropharmacological, neuroanatomic, and biochemical data (Cloninger 1987, 1994b) and on studies of the phylogeny of learning abilities (Cloninger 1994a), which are briefly described here.

Novelty seeking is characterized by exhilaration and exploration in response to novel stimuli, approach to signals of reward, active avoidance of conditioned signals of punishment, and escape from unconditioned punishment. All four of these behaviors are hypothesized to covary as part of one heritable

Table 3–5. Four dissociable brain systems influencing stimulus-response patterns underlying temperament

Brain system (related personality dimension)	Principal neuromodulators	Relevant stimuli	Behavioral response
Behavioral activation (novelty seeking)	Dopamine	Novelty CS of reward CS or UCS of relief of monotony or punishment	Exploratory pursuit Appetive approach Active avoidance, escape
Behavioral inhibition (harm avoidance)	GABA Serotonin (dorsal raphe)	Aversive conditioning (pairing CS and UCS) Conditioned signals for punishment, novelty, or frustrative nonreward	Formation of aversive CS Passive avoidance, extinction
Social attachment (reward dependence)	Norepinephrine Serotonin (median raphe)	Reward conditioning (pairing CS and UCS)	Formation of appetitive CS
Partial reinforcement (persistence)	Glutamate Serotonin (dorsal raphe)	Intermittent reinforcement	Resistance to extinction

Note. CS, conditioned signals; UCS, unconditioned signals; GABA, γ-aminobutyric acid.
Source. Adapted from Cloninger 1987, 1994; Deakin 1996.

system of learning, just as there is strong covariation among different components of novelty seeking, including thrill seeking (i.e., exploration of novelty); impulsive, extravagant spending (i.e., approach to signals of reward); quick-tempered argumentation (i.e., active avoidance); and running away from home (i.e., escape). Mesolimbic and mesofrontal dopaminergic projections have been shown to play a crucial role in incentive activation of each aspect of novelty seeking (Cloninger 1987). Dopamine-depleting lesions in the nucleus accumbens or the ventral tegmentum lead to neglect of novel environmental stimuli and reduce both spontaneous activity and investigative behavior. Behavioral activation by dopaminergic agonists depends on the integrity of the nucleus accumbens but not the caudate nucleus. In human studies, individuals at risk for Parkinson's disease have low premorbid scores in novelty seeking but not other dimensions of personality (Menza et al. 1995), supporting the importance of dopamine in incentive activation of pleasurable behavior. The initiation and frequency of hyperactivity, binge eating, sexual hedonism, drinking, smoking, and other substance abuse, especially of stimulants, are each associated with high scores in novelty seeking (Bardo et al. 1996; Downey et al. 1996; Fergusson and Lynskey 1996; Howard et al. 1996). Other supporting neurophysiological, neuroanatomic, and biochemical data are reviewed elsewhere (Bardo et al. 1996; Cloninger 1987, 1994b).

Harm avoidance is a heritable tendency to be worried, fearful, shy, and fatigable (Table 3–2). In terms of procedural learning (Table 3–4), harm-avoidant individuals are hypothesized to be predisposed to form conditioned signals of punishment and frustrative nonreward (i.e., they worry and are easily frightened) and to be sensitive to passive avoidance learning, which is the inhibition of activity in response to such conditioned signals. In other words, individuals who are highly harm avoidant respond intensely to conditioned aversive signals (i.e., they are easily inhibited, shy, and fatigable). Ascending serotonergic projections from the dorsal raphe nuclei to the substantia nigra inhibit nigrostriatal dopaminergic neurons and are essential for conditioned inhibition of activity by signals of punishment and frustrative nonreward (Cloninger 1987; Deakin and Graeff 1991). Benzodiazepines disinhibit passive avoidance conditioning by γ-aminobutyric acid (GABA)-ergic inhibition of serotonergic neurons originating in the dorsal raphe nuclei (Sepinwall and Cook 1980; Stein 1981). The anterior serotonergic cells in the dorsal raphe nucleus intermingle with the dopaminergic cells of the ventral tegmental area, and both groups innervate the same structures (i.e., basal ganglia, accumbens, and amygdala), providing opposing dopaminergic-serotonergic influences in the modulation of approach and avoidance behavior. The anterior serotonergic projections from the dorsal raphe to striatum, accumbens, amygdala, and frontal cortex are usually associated with 5-HT$_2$ receptors (Deakin and Graeff 1991). Individuals who score high in both harm avoidance and novelty seeking are expected to have frequent approach-avoidance conflicts, as seen in cycles of bingeing and purging in bulimia (Cloninger 1994b). More generally, excessive behavioral inhibition (i.e., high harm avoidance) predisposes individuals to anxiety, depression, and low self-esteem. Effective antidepressant treatment lowers scores in harm avoidance, but higher scores in harm avoidance predict poorer responses to antidepressants, including tricyclics and selective serotonin reuptake inhibitors (SSRIs) (Joffe et al. 1993; Joyce et al. 1994; Tome et al. 1997).

Reward dependence is hypothesized to be a heritable predisposition for facility in the development of conditioned signals of reward, particularly social cues. Noradrenergic projections from the locus coeruleus and serotonergic projections from the median raphe are proposed to influence such reward conditioning (Table 3–4). In animals, stimulation of the noradrenergic locus coeruleus or its dorsal bundle or direct application of norepinephrine decreases the firing rate of terminal neurons and increases their sensitivity to other afferents, so that targeted stimuli can stand out from nontargeted stimuli (Segal and Bloom 1976). In humans, short-term reduction of norepinephrine release by acute infusion of the α$_2$ presynaptic agonist clonidine selectively impairs paired-associate learning, particularly the acquisition of novel associations (Frith et al. 1985). The noradrenergic locus coeruleus is located at the same posterior level of the brain stem as the serotonergic median raphe, and both of these posterior monoamine cells innervate structures important to the formation of paired associations, such as the thalamus, neocortex, and hippocampus (Deakin 1996). Whereas 5-HT_{2a} receptors in the frontal cortex are innervated particularly by projections from the dorsal raphe, the terminals of the median raphe innervate 5-HT_{1a} receptors in the anterior and medial temporal lobe. Neurophysiological studies show that the anterior temporal lobe is specialized to decode social signals, such as facial images and social gestures. Consequently, individuals high in reward dependence are expected to be particularly sensitive in their social communication, whereas those low in reward dependence are expected to be socially aloof.

Persistence is a fourth heritable dimension of temperament. Persistent individuals are eager, ambitious, and determined overachievers. Persistence can be measured objectively by the partial reinforcement extinction effect (PREE), in which persistent individuals are more resistant to the extinction of previously intermittently rewarded behavior than other individuals who have been continuously reinforced. Originally (Cloninger 1987), I proposed that persistence was a component of reward dependence because animal experiments suggested that lesions of the dorsal noradrenergic bundle lead to increased resistance to extinction of previously rewarded behavior (Mason and Iversen 1979). However, animal studies of the dorsal bundle extinction effect were found to be nonreproducible. Also, human studies showed that persistence was weakly and inconsistently correlated with reward dependence (Cloninger et al. 1993) and that it was independently inherited (Stallings et al. 1996). Recent work in rodents showed that the integrity of the PREE depends on projections from the hippocampal subiculum to the nucleus accumbens (Tai et al. 1991). This glutaminergic projection may be considered as a short circuit from the behavioral inhibition system to the behavioral activation system, thereby converting a conditioned signal of punishment into a conditioned signal of anticipated reward. This connection is probably disrupted in humans by lesions of the orbitomedial cortex that may have a specific antipersistence effect of therapeutic benefit to some severely obsessive-compulsive patients (Cloninger 1994b). Bilateral cingulotomy, which reduces harm avoidance only, is less effective in reducing persistent compulsive behavior than cingulotomy combined with orbitomedial lesions (Hay et al. 1993).

Genomewide Scan for Loci Linked to Human Personality

Recently the first genomewide scan of human temperament has been carried out using the TPQ in a sample of 758 sibling pairs in 177 nuclear families (Cloninger et al. 1997, in press). The families were ascertained because of a high density of alcoholism as part of the Collaborative Study of the Genetics of Alcoholism (Cloninger et al., in press). Each member of these families completed the TPQ and was genotyped with 291 polymorphic markers spaced at regular intervals along all of the human chromosomes. The total length of the human chromosomes is estimated at around 3.7 M, or 3,700 cM, so the average interval between the 291 successive markers was 13 cM. Such a moderately dense map allows effective screening to detect linkage between each trait and genetic loci. Linkage is shown when differences between family members in each trait are correlated with measures of the genetic identity of family members at specific loci along each chromosome. Using variance component analysis, we also estimated the amount of variance in each trait explained by genetic variation at different loci. As summarized in Table 3–6, we detected significant linkage between TPQ harm avoidance and a genetic locus on the short arm of chromosome 8 (more specifically, region 8p21–23), in the vicinity of marker *D8S1106*, which accounted for most of the additive genetic variance (20%–30%) in harm avoidance in this sample. Multiplicative gene-gene (epistatic) interactions with other genes on chromosome 21q21–22.1, and possibly 18p and 20p, explained most of the total variance in harm avoidance (54%–66%) and nearly all of its heritable variance.

Most of the heritable variation in each of the TPQ traits was attributable to a different set of such epistatic loci, confirming

Table 3–6. Multilocus epistatic interactions in linkage analysis of human personality

Temperament trait	Locus	lod score	P	Explained variance
Harm avoidance	8:17	5.1	7×10^{-6}	66%
	21:62			
Reward dependence	2:4	5.3	.0005	53%
	2:116			
	16:15			
Novelty seeking	10:88	2.8	.02	50%
	15:65			
Persistence	2:158	2.5	.01	45%
	3:220			

Source. Cloninger et al. 1997, in press.

the genetic independence of the four temperament dimensions inferred from twin studies (Stallings et al. 1996). Genomewide scans such as this are most helpful in detecting sets of epistatic genes or individual genes with moderately large effects. Such scans may be insensitive to smaller contributions that may be detectable by association with a specific candidate gene. We plan to type additional flanking markers and candidate genes in the regions identified as promising in this initial linkage scan, such as genes for the kainate-sensitive subunit of glutamate receptor 5 on 21q22.1. This glutamate receptor subtype is primarily expressed in the CA3 region of the hippocampus, which has crucial interactions with serotonin receptors in the regulation of anxiety and related behaviors including trembling (Isaacson and Lanthorn 1981).

Psychobiological Correlates of Temperament and Character

Reported Psychobiological Correlates of Harm Avoidance

Over the past decade extensive information has been obtained by many independent investigators to test the theoretical predictions I have made about the psychobiology of each of the seven dimensions of personality. Neuroanatomic, neuropsychological, neurochemical, and neurogenetic candidate gene studies about harm avoidance are summarized in Table 3–7.

Neuropsychological studies confirm that harm avoidance is associated with individual differences in classical aversive conditioning, whereas other dimensions of personality are uncorrelated (Corr et al. 1995a). Harm avoidance, and not other dimensions of temperament, is also replicably associated with potentiation of the startle responses to air puffs to the eyelids, which is an aversive stimulus (Corr et al. 1995b, 1997). There have been no direct tests of passive avoidant learning with the TPQ personality variables, but other neuropsychological tests confirm effects involving behavioral inhibition. For example, harm avoidance is associated with the Posner validity effect. The Posner task uses a detection reaction time paradigm with discrete presentation of simple visual stimuli in the periphery. Cues that correctly direct attention to the spatial location where the target stimulus will appear are called valid cues, whereas those that direct attention to incorrect locations are called invalid cues. In three large samples of healthy college students, individuals who are higher in harm avoidance showed greater slowing of their reactions after invalid cues, or less benefit from valid cues, than others ($r = .28, .30, .38$ in each study) (Cloninger et al. 1994).

Positron-emission tomography (PET) at the National Institute of Mental Health (NIMH) with 18-fluorodeoxyglucose in 31 healthy adult volunteers who took the TPQ confirmed that harm avoidance was associated with increased activity in the anterior paralimbic circuit, specifically the right amygdala and insula, the right orbitofrontal cortex, and the left medial prefrontal cortex (M. S. George, T. A. Kimbrell, M. Willis, et al., written communication, May 1996). This activation pattern corresponds well to the 5-HT$_2$ terminal projections of the dorsal raphe. However, 5-HT$_2$ has been measured in platelets only (see Table 3–7).

Higher plasma GABA levels have been correlated with low harm avoidance (Table 3–7). Plasma GABA has also been correlated with other measures of anxiety proneness and correlates highly with brain GABA levels (Cowley et al. 1996). Finally, a gene on chromosome 17q12 that regulates the expression of the

Table 3–7. Reported psychobiological correlates of harm avoidance

Variable	Effect	Subjects	Reference
Neuroanatomy (PET)			
Medial prefrontal (L)	++ activity	Healthy subjects	George et al. 1996
Anterior paralimbic (R)	++ activity	Healthy subjects	
Neuropsychology			
Aversive conditioning	Associative pairing ($r = .4$)	Healthy subjects	Corr et al. 1995a
Eyeblink startle reflex	Potentiation (effect size 1.9)	Healthy subjects	Corr et al. 1995b, 1997
Posner validity effect	Slower ($r = .3$)	Healthy subjects	Swanson et al. 1994
Spatial delayed response	Better delay ($r = .5$)	Healthy subjects	Fleming et al. 1995
		p-Amphetamine	
Neurochemistry			
Platelet 5-HT$_2$ receptor	Fewer ($r = -.6$)	Depressed subjects	Nelson et al. 1996
Plasma GABA	Lower ($r = -.5$)	Healthy subjects and sons of alcoholic patients	Cowley et al. 1996
Neurogenetics			
5-HT transporter promoter	.3 effect size	Healthy subjects	Lesch et al. 1996
	.5 effect size	Families	Lesch et al. 1996
	.5 effect size	Elderly subjects	Ricketts et al. (in press)
	.9 effect size	Young women	Nakamura et al. 1997
	No effect	Healthy subjects	Ball et al. 1997
	No effect	Healthy subjects	Ebstein et al. 1997

Note. PET, positron-emission tomography; L, left; R, right; GABA, γ-aminobutyric acid.

serotonin transporter has been found to account for 4%–9% of the total variance in harm avoidance; this effect has been observed in four of the six studies shown in Table 3–7. These findings support a role for both GABA and serotonergic projections from the dorsal raphe underlying individual differences in behavioral inhibition as measured by the trait of harm avoidance.

Reported Psychobiological Correlates of Novelty Seeking

The psychobiological correlates reported for novelty seeking are summarized in Table 3–8. High scores are associated with increased metabolic activity on PET in the cingulate cortex and left caudate (M. S. George, T. A. Kimbrell, M. Willis, et al., written communication, May 1996; Menza et al. 1995). In addition, high novelty seeking is associated with decreased activity in the left medial prefrontal cortex, which is exactly the same region associated with increased activity in individuals scoring high in harm avoidance. This finding suggests that the medial prefrontal cortex may be an important site in the processing of approach-avoidance conflicts.

Evoked potential studies of stimulus intensity dependence confirm that novelty seeking is associated with augmentation of stimulus intensity, particularly with novel stimuli (Juckel et al. 1995). Novelty seekers are also sensitive to both sedatives and stimulants: they are easily oversedated by benzodiazepines (Cowley et al. 1993) and overstimulated by amphetamines, leading to deterioration in their information processing (Fleming et al. 1995). Their reaction times are slow to neutral stimuli (Corr et al. 1995a).

The association of increased striatal activity with high novelty seeking is more specifically associated with higher density of the dopamine transporter in alcoholic patients (Tiihonen et al. 1995), suggesting that novelty seeking involves increased reuptake of dopamine at presynaptic terminals, thereby requiring extraordinary stimulation to maintain optimal levels of postsynaptic dopaminergic stimulation. Novelty seeking leads to various pleasure-seeking behaviors, including cigarette smoking, which may explain the frequent observation of low platelet monoamine oxidase (MAO) B activity because cigarette smoking has the effect of inhibiting MAO B activity in platelets and in brain (Fowler et al. 1996).

Studies of candidate genes involved in dopamine neurotransmission (e.g., dopamine transporter and D4DR) have provided evidence of association with novelty seeking and no other dimension of temperament. The dopamine transporter, which is responsible for presynaptic reuptake of dopamine and a major site of action of drugs including stimulants such as methylphenidate and the antidepressant bupropion, is encoded by locus SLC6A3 (alias DAT1) on chromosome 5p (Gelernter et al. 1995). A polymorphism of this gene locus is associated with attention-deficit disorder (Cook et al. 1995; Gill et al. 1997) and other disorders related to variation in novelty seeking (Blum et al. 1997; Comings et al. 1996). Novelty seeking has not been measured directly in these studies, and the results are not consistent even when novelty seeking is measured (see Table 3–8). This result is not surprising given the evidence of epistatic (nonlinear) interactions among multiple loci in our genomewide linkage scan. Additional support for the initial reports of linkage and association between the D4DR locus and novelty seeking comes from several reports confirming the allelic association between the exon III polymorphism of D4DR with attention-deficit/hyperactivity disorder (LaHoste et al. 1996) and with opioid dependence (Kotler et al. 1997), which are both associated with high degrees of novelty seeking.

Reported Psychobiological Correlates of Reward Dependence

The psychobiological correlates reported about reward dependence are summarized in Table 3–9. As predicted, reward dependence is associated with individual differences in the formation of conditioned signals of reward (Corr et al. 1995a). This finding is also supported by its association with individual dif-

Table 3–8. Reported psychobiological correlates of novelty seeking

Variable	Effect	Subjects	Reference
Neuroanatomy (PET)			
Prefrontal (L)	− − activity	Healthy subjects	George et al. 1996
Cingulate	+ + activity	Healthy subjects	
Caudate (L)	+ + activity	Healthy subjects	
Caudate (L)	+ + dopamine uptake	Parkinson's disease patients	Menza et al. 1995
Neuropsychology			
Reaction time	Slower ($r = -.4$) if not reinforced	Healthy subjects	Corr et al. 1995a
Stimulus intensity (N_1/P_2 ERP)	Augments novelty ($r = .5$)	Healthy subjects	Juckel et al. 1995
Sedation threshold (saccades p-diazapam)	Lower to sedation ($r = -.3$)	GAD and healthy subjects	Cowley et al. 1993
Rey word list memory	Deteriorates p-amphetamine ($r = .6$)	Healthy subjects	Fleming et al. 1995
Neurochemistry			
Striatal dopamine transporter	Higher density (SPECT)	Alcoholic patients	Tiihonen et al. 1995
Platelet MAO B	Lower activity		
	($r = -.5$)	Healthy subjects	Sullivan et al. 1990
	($r = -.3$)	Alcoholic patients	Sullivan et al. 1990
	($r = -.5$)	Alcoholic patients' sons	Howard et al. 1996
	($r = -.6$)	Abstinent alcoholic patients	Rommelspacher et al. 1994

Neurogenetics

Dopamine receptor D_4	.3 effect size	Healthy subjects	Ebstein et al. 1996
	.4 effect size	Healthy subjects	Benjamin et al. 1996
	.4 effect size	Families	Benjamin et al. 1996
	Effect with NS_1	Young women	Ono et al. 1997
	No effect	Alcoholic and healthy subjects	Malhotra et al. 1997
	No effect	Alcoholic and healthy subjects	Sander et al. (in press)
Dopamine transporter	No effect	Healthy subjects	Sullivan et al. 1997
	.4 effect size	ADHD subjects	Cook et al. 1995
	No effect	Healthy subjects	Sullivan et al. 1997

Note. PET, positron-emission tomography; L, left; ADHD, attention-deficit/hyperactivity disorder; MAO, monoamine oxidase; ERP, early receptor potential; SPECT, single photon emission computed tomography.

Table 3–9. Reported psychobiological correlates of reward dependence

Variable	Effect	Subjects	Reference
Neuroanatomy (PET)			
Thalamus	++ activity	Healthy subjects	George et al. 1996
Neuropsychology			
Reward conditioning	Associative pairing ($r = .3$)	Healthy subjects	Corr et al. 1995a
Paired associates	Better learning ($r = .5$)	Healthy subjects	Fleming et al. 1995
Posner validity effect	Faster learning ($r = -.4$)	Healthy subjects	Swanson et al. 1994
Neurochemistry			
Urinary MHPG	Less excretion ($r = -.4$)	Alcoholic patients	Garvey et al. 1996
Urinary harman	Greater excretion ($r = .7$)	Alcoholic patients	Wodarz et al. 1996
Neurogenetics			
5-HT$_{2c}$ receptor	2.0 effect size	Healthy subjects	Ebstein et al. 1997

Note. PET, positron-emission tomography; MHPG, 3-methoxy-4-hydroxyphenylglycol.

ferences in paired-associate learning under placebo conditions (Cloninger et al. 1994; Fleming et al. 1995).

High reward dependence is associated with increased activity in the thalamus (George et al. 1996), which is consistent with Deakin's (1996) proposal about the importance of serotonergic projections to the thalamus from the median raphe in the modulation of social communication. This association is further supported by the finding of low levels of urinary 3-methoxy-4-hydroxyphenylglycol (MHPG) in alcoholic patients with high reward dependence (Garvey et al. 1996). Other studies of alcoholic patients in Germany have observed higher levels of the β-carboline harman, which results from the interaction of indoleamines and acetaldehyde in alcoholic patients (Wodarz et al. 1996).

Ebstein et al. (1997b) have reported a substantial allelic association between a polymorphism at the 5-HT_{2c} receptor locus and both reward dependence and persistence. These effects were further facilitated by interactions with *D4DR* and *D3DR* (Ebstein et al. 1997b). No work has been reported about the 5-HT_1 receptor and any temperament dimension, but such investigation may be worthwhile as a test of Deakin's prediction about these receptors and social learning.

Reported Psychobiological Correlates of Persistence

The reported correlates of persistence are summarized in Table 3–10. Much less work is available about persistence than about the other dimensions, possibly because it has been distinguished as an independently inherited dimension only since 1993 (Cloninger et al. 1993). Neuropsychological studies confirm that individuals high in persistence qualities make more effort to learn without reinforcement (Cloninger et al. 1994; Fleming et al. 1995). In laboratory gambling tasks, highly persistent individuals are also more perseverative; that is, they exhibit the "gambler's fallacy" by maintaining the same bet size despite repeated losses.

Table 3–10. Reported psychobiological correlates of persistence

Variable	Effect	Subjects	Reference
Neuroanatomy			
Orbitomedial cortex	Disconnection reduces perseveration	Obsessive patients	Hay et al. 1993 Cloninger 1994
Neuropsychology			
Bet size despite loss in gambling task	Perseveration ($r = .4$)	Healthy subjects	Christodoulou et al. 1995
Rey word list learning	Learning without reinforcement ($r = .5$)	Healthy subjects	Fleming et al. 1995 Cloninger et al. 1994
Neurochemistry			
Glutaminergic connection Subiculum to nucleus accumbens	Essential for PREE[a]	Rats	Tai et al. 1991
Neurogenetics			
5-HT$_{2c}$ receptor	2.0 effect size	Healthy subjects	Ebstein et al. 1997

[a] Partial reinforcement extinction effect (PREE) is persistence or increased resistance to extinction following intermittent reinforcement.

Reported Psychobiological Correlates of Character

The distinction between temperament and character would be much clearer if an objective test could discriminate character traits from temperament traits. Recently, Vedeniapin et al. (1997) observed that TCI self-directedness is moderately correlated with the evoked potential P300 ($r = .3$, $P = .02$) in parietal regions of 56 healthy subjects (Table 3–11). P300 was not correlated with other dimensions of personality, and the correlation with self-directedness was unchanged by controlling for harm avoidance and other temperament and character dimensions. Likewise, contingent negative variation was moderately correlated with TCI cooperativeness and to a lesser degree with TCI self-transcendence but not with self-directedness or any temperament dimension.

Conclusions

Over the past decade extensive information has been obtained by many independent investigators that provides empirical tests of the theoretical model for human personality that I have described. These tests have been facilitated by the widespread availability of brief, reliable, quantitative self-report inventories for measuring temperament (TPQ) and character (TCI). Avail-

Table 3–11. Relation of character traits to psychobiological differences in event-related potentials in parietal leads of healthy adult individuals

	Correlation with	
Character trait	P300	CNV
Self-directedness	+.31 ($P = .023$)	−.26 (NS)
Cooperativeness	+.14 (NS)	−.34 ($P = .035$)
Self-transcendence	+.06 (NS)	−.32 ($P = .048$)

Note. P300 is the averaged amplitudes of P300 across parietal leads (P3, Pz, P4) in 56 subjects; CNV is early contingent negative variation across parietal leads (P3, Pz, P4) in 37 subjects. All correlations controlled for age; correlations of P300 were controlled for other character traits.
Source. Vedeniapin et al. 1997.

able data are generally supportive of the seven-factor model, including the major domains of temperament and character and the subdivisions of each of these domains.

There has been a remarkable degree of confirmation of theoretical predictions originally made in 1987 with the empirical findings about neuroanatomy, neuropsychology, neurochemistry, and neurogenetics a decade later. The original emphasis on the importance of dopaminergic neuromodulation in novelty seeking, serotonergic neuromodulation from the dorsal raphe in harm avoidance, and noradrenergic influences in reward dependence has generally been supported. However, persistence has emerged as a fourth heritable dimension with distinct psychobiological correlates, and three dimensions of character have been distinguished from those of temperament. Also, the psychobiology of each system involves interactions among multiple genes and multiple neurotransmitter systems.

The seven-factor model of personality provides a useful framework for providing a fuller understanding of the psychobiology of multiple dimensions of human personality. It can account for diagnostic clusters and categories in terms of multidimensional profiles that are relatively stable developmentally, as well as providing quantitative measures of use in both psychobiological research and clinical practice. Of great practical significance are the recent replications of the finding that the seven-factor model of personality predicts individual differences in response to antidepressants (Joffe et al. 1993; Joyce et al. 1994; Tome et al. 1997). This finding allows the emerging understanding of the psychobiology of personality to guide clinical practice by informing the choice of different drugs and drug combinations along with psychotherapy (Cloninger and Svrakic 1997; Tome et al. 1997).

Another point needs to be made before closing. My work and the work of others (Siever and Davis 1991) have attempted to correlate different dimensions of behavior and personality with different neurotransmitter systems. The amount of work undertaken since each of these theories was proposed between 7 and 10 years ago is remarkable (Cloninger 1987; Cloninger et al. 1993; Siever and Davis 1991). On the one hand, the amount of work may reflect the strong desire and need for a biological theory of personality and the pathology of personality. On the other hand, and humbly speaking, the amount of work may reflect the degree to which the proposed theories resonate with clinical and research intuition. But for our purposes here, perhaps the strongest point that should be made reflects the idea that more and more sophisticated methods and methodologies are being applied in ever-increasing frequency in an attempt to unravel the biological underpinnings of the behaviors that constitute personality and its disorders.

References

American Psychiatric Association: Diagnostic and Statistical Manual of Mental Disorders, 4th Edition. Washington, DC, American Psychiatric Association, 1994

Ball D, Hill L, Freeman B, et al: The serotonin transporter gene and peer-rated neuroticism. Neuroreport 8:1301–1304, 1997

Bardo MT, Donohew RL, Harrington NG: Psychobiology of novelty seeking and drug seeking behavior. Behav Brain Res 77:23–43, 1996

Bayon C, Hill K, Svrakic DM, et al: Dimensional assessment of personality in an outpatient sample: relations of the systems of Millon and Cloninger. J Psychiatr Res 30:341–352, 1996

Benjamin J, Li L, Patterson C, et al: Population and familial association between the D_4 dopamine receptor and measures of novelty seeking. Nat Genet 12:81–84, 1996

Blum K, Braverman ER, Wu S, et al: Association of polymorphisms of dopamine D_2 receptor (DRD2) and dopamine transporter (DAT1) with schizoid/avoidant behaviors (SAB). Molecular Psychiatry 2:239–246, 1997

Christodoulou C, Rosen JJ, Janal MN, et al: Personality differences in patterns of risk taking while gambling. Psychol Rep 76:1307–1314, 1995

Cloninger CR: A unified biosocial theory of personality and its role in the development of anxiety states. Psychiatr Dev 3:167–226, 1986

Cloninger CR: A systematic method for clinical description and classification of personality variants. Arch Gen Psychiatry 44:579–588, 1987

Cloninger CR: Genetic structure of personality and learning: a phylogenetic structure. Clin Genet 46:124–137, 1994a

Cloninger CR: Temperament and personality. Curr Opin Neurobiol 4:266–273, 1994b

Cloninger CR: The psychobiological regulation of social cooperation. Nat Med 1:623–625, 1995

Cloninger CR, Svrakic DM: Integrative psychobiological approach to psychiatric assessment and treatment. Psychiatry 60:120–141, 1997

Cloninger CR, Svrakic DM, Pryzbeck TR: A psychobiological model of temperament and characters. Arch Gen Psychiatry 50:975–990, 1993

Cloninger CR, Pryzbeck TR, Svrakic DM, et al: The Temperament and Character Inventory (TCI): A Guide to Its Development and Use. St. Louis, MO, Washington University Center for Psychobiology of Personality, 1994

Cloninger CR, Van Eerdewegh P, Goate A, et al: Epistatic quantitative trait loci in a genome-wide scan of human personality by the Collaborative Study of the Genetics of Alcoholism. Paper presented at the International Society of Psychiatric Genetics, Sante Fe, NM, October 1997

Cloninger CR, Van Eerdewegh P, Goate A, et al: Anxiety proneness linked to epistatic loci in genome scan of human personality traits. Am J Med Genet (in press)

Comings DE, Wu S, Chiu C, et al: Polygenic inheritance of Tourette syndrome, stuttering, attention deficit hyperactivity, conduct, and oppositional defiant disorder. Am J Med Genet 67:264–288, 1996

Cook EH Jr, Stein MA, Krasowski MD, et al: Association of attention deficit disorder and the dopamine transporter gene. Am J Hum Genet 56:993–998, 1995

Corr PJ, Pickering AD, Gray JA: Personality and reinforcement in associative and instrumental learning. Personality and Individual Differences 19:47–71, 1995a

Corr PJ, Wilson GD, Fotiadou M, et al: Personality and affective modulation of the startle reflex. Personality and Individual Differences 19:543–553, 1995b

Corr PJ, Kumari V, Wilson GD, et al: Harm avoidance and affective modulation of the startle reflex: a replication. Personality and Individual Differences 22:591–593, 1997

Cowley DS, Roy-Byrne PP, Greenblatt DJ, et al: Personality and benzodiazepine sensitivity in anxious patients and control subjects. Psychiatry Res 47:151–162, 1993

Cowley DS, Roy-Byrne PP, Greenblatt DJ, et al: Effect of diazepam on plasma gamma-aminobutyric acid in sons of alcoholic fathers. Alcohol Clin Exp Res 20:343–347, 1996

Deakin JFW: 5-HT, antidepressant drugs, and the psychosocial origins of depression. Journal of Psychopharmacology 10:31–38, 1996

Deakin JFW, Graeff FG: 5-HT and mechanisms of defence. Journal of Psychopharmacology 5:305–315, 1991

Downey KK, Pomerleau CS, Pomerleau OF: Personality differences related to smoking and adult attention deficit hyperactivity disorder. J Subst Abuse 8:129–135, 1996

Ebstein RP, Novick O, Umansky R, et al: Dopamine D_4 receptor *(D4DR)* exon III polymorphism associated with the human personality trait of novelty seeking. Nat Genet 12:78–80, 1996

Ebstein RP, Gritsenko I, Nemanov L, et al: No association between the serotonin transporter gene regulatory region polymorphism and the Tridimensional Personality Questionnaire (TPQ) temperament of harm avoidance. Molecular Psychiatry 2:224–226, 1997a

Ebstein RP, Segman R, Benjamin J, et al: 5-HT_{2C} *(HTR2C)* serotonin receptor gene polymorphism associated with the human personality trait of reward dependence: interaction with dopamine D_4 receptor *(D4DR)* and dopamine D_3 receptor *(D3DR)* polymorphisms. Am J Med Genet 74:65–72, 1997b

Fergusson DM, Lynskey MT: Alcohol misuse and adolescent sexual behaviors and risk taking. Pediatrics 98:91–96, 1996

Fleming K, Bigelow LB, Weinberger DR, et al: Neuropsychological effects of amphetamine may correlate with personality characteristics. Psychopharmacol Bull 31:358–362, 1995

Fowler JS, Volkow ND, Wang G-J, et al: Inhibition of monoamine oxidase B in the brains of smokers. Nature 379:733–736, 1996

Frith CD, Dowdy J, Ferrier IN, et al: Selective impairment of paired associate learning after administration of a centrally-acting adrenergic agonist (clonidine). Psychopharmacology 87:490–493, 1985

Garvey MJ, Noyes R Jr, Cook B, et al: Preliminary confirmation of the proposed link between reward-dependence traits and norepinephrine. Psychiatry Res 65:61–64, 1996

Gelernter J, Vandenbergh D, Kruger SD, et al: The dopamine transporter protein gene *(SLC6A3)*: primary linkage mapping and linkage studies in Tourette syndrome. Genomics 30:459–463, 1995

Gill M, Daly G, Heron S, et al: Confirmation of association between attention deficit hyperactivity disorder and a dopamine transporter polymorphism. Molecular Psychiatry 2:311–313, 1997

Goldman RG, Skodal AE, McGrath PJ, et al: Tridimensional Personality Questionnaire and DSM-III-R personality traits. Am J Psychiatry 151:274–276, 1994

Goldsmith HH, Buss AH, Plomin R, et al: What is temperament? four approaches. Child Dev 58:505–529, 1987

Hay P, Sachdev P, Cummings S, et al: Treatment of obsessive-compulsive disorder by psychosurgery. Acta Psychiatr Scand 87:197–207, 1993

Howard MO, Cowley DS, Roy-Byrne PP, et al: Tridimensional personality traits in sons of alcoholic and nonalcoholic fathers. Alcohol Clin Exp Res 20:445–448, 1996

Isaacson RL, Lanthorn TH: Hippocampal involvement in the pharmacological induction of withdrawal-like behaviors. Federation Proceedings 40:1508–1512, 1981

Joffe RT, Bagby RM, Levitt AJ, et al: The Tridimensional Personality Questionnaire in major depression. Am J Psychiatry 150:959–960, 1993

Joyce PR, Mulder RT, Cloninger CR: Temperament predicts clomipramine and desipramine response in major depression. J Affective Disord 30:35–46, 1994

Juckel G, Schmidt LG, Rommelspacher H, et al: The Tridimensional Personality Questionnaire and the intensity dependence of auditory evoked dipole source activity. Biol Psychiatry 37:311–317, 1995

Kant I: Anthropology From a Pragmatic Point of View (1798). Translated by Gregor MJ. The Hague, Martinus Nijhoff, 1974

Kotler M, Cohen H, Segman R, et al: Excess dopamine D_4 receptor (D4DR) exon III seven repeat allele in opioid-dependent subjects. Molecular Psychiatry 2:251–254, 1997

LaHoste GJ, Swanson JM, Wigal SB, et al: Dopamine D_4 receptor gene polymorphism is associated with attention deficit hyperactivity disorder. Molecular Psychiatry 1:121–124, 1996

Lesch KP, Bengal D, Heils A, et al: Association of anxiety-related traits with a polymorphism in the serotonin transporter gene regulatory region. Science 274:1527–1531, 1996

Malhotra AK, Virkkunen M, Rooney W, et al: The association between the dopamine D_4 receptor (D4DR) 16 amino acid repeat polymorphism and novelty seeking. Molecular Psychiatry 1:388–391, 1996

Mason ST, Iversen ST: Theories of the dorsal bundle extinction effect. Brain Res Rev 1:107–137, 1979

Menza MA, Mark MH, Burn DJ, et al: Psychiatric correlates of ^{18}F-dopa striatal uptake: results of positron emission tomography in Parkinson's disease. J Neuropsychiatry Clin Neurosci 7:176–179, 1995

Nagoshi CT, Walter D, Muntaner C, et al: Validation of the Tridimensional Personality Questionnaire in a sample of male drug users. Personality and Individual Differences 13:401–409, 1992

Nakamura T, Muramatsu T, Ono Y, et al: Serotonin transporter gene regulatory region polymorphism and anxiety-related traits in the Japanese. Am J Med Genet 74:544–545, 1997

Nelson EC, Cloninger CR, Przybeck TR, et al: Platelet serotonergic markers and Tridimensional Personality Questionnaire measures in a clinical sample. Biol Psychiatry 40:271–278, 1996

Ono Y, Manki H, Yoshimura K, et al: Association between dopamine D_4 receptor (D4DR) exon III polymorphism and novelty seeking in Japanese subjects. Am J Med Genet (in press)

Ricketts MH, Hamer RM, Sage JI, et al: Association of a serotonin transporter gene promoter polymorphism with harm avoidance behavior in an elderly population. Psychiatr Genet (in press)

Rommelspacher H, May T, Dufeu P, et al: Longitudinal observations of monoamine oxidase B in alcoholics: differentiation of marker characteristics. Alcohol Clin Exp Res 18:1322–1329, 1994

Sander T, Harms H, Dufeu P, et al: Dopamine D_4 receptor exon III alleles and variation of novelty seeking in alcoholics. Am J Med Genet (in press)

Segal M, Bloom FE: The action of norepinephrine in the rat hippocampus, IV: the effects of locus coeruleus stimulation on evoked hippocampal unit activity. Brain Res 107:513–525, 1976

Sepinwall J, Cook L: Mechanism of action of the benzodiazepines: behavioral aspects. Federation Proceedings 39:3021–3031, 1980

Siever LJ, Davis L: A psychobiological perspective on the personality disorders. Am J Psychiatry 148:1647–1658, 1991

Stallings MC, Hewitt JK, Cloninger CR, et al: Genetic and environmental structure of the Tridimensional Personality Questionnaire: three or four temperament dimensions? J Pers Soc Psychol 70:127–140, 1996

Stein L: Behavioral pharmacology of benzodiazepines, in Anxiety: New Research and Changing Concepts. Edited by Klein DF, Rabkin J. New York, Raven, 1981, pp 201–214

Sullivan PF, Fifield WJ, Kennedy MA, et al: No association between novelty seeking and the type 4 dopamine receptor gene (DRD4) in two New Zealand samples. Am J Psychiatry (in press [a])

Sullivan PF, Fifield WJ, Kennedy MA, et al: Novelty seeking and a dopamine transporter gene polymorphism (DAT1). Biol Psychiatry (in press [b])

Svrakic DM, Whitehead C, Przybeck TR, et al: Differential diagnosis of personality disorders by the seven factor model of temperament and character. Arch Gen Psychiatry 50:991–999, 1993

Svrakic NM, Svrakic DM, Cloninger CR: A general quantitative theory of personality development: fundamentals of a self-organizing psychobiological complex. Development and Psychopathology 8:247–272, 1996

Swanson JM, Wigal T, Conboy MS, et al: Use of MEL and dBASE programs in large sample experiments: correlation of scores on Cloninger's personality dimensions with performance measures on Posner's laboratory test of attention, in TCI: Guide to Its Development and Use. Edited by Cloninger CR, Przybeck TR, Svrakic DM, et al. St. Louis, MO, Washington University Center for Psychobiology, 1994, pp 141–143

Tai CT, Clark AJM, Feldon J, et al: Electrolytic lesions of the nucleus accumbens in rats which abolish the PREE enhance the locomotor response to amphetamine. Exp Brain Res 86:333–340, 1991

Tiihonen J, Kuikka J, Bergstrom K, et al: Altered striatal dopamine reuptake site densities in habitually violent and non-violent alcoholics. Nat Med 1:654–657, 1995

Tome MB, Cloninger CR, Watson JP, et al: Serotonergic autoreceptor blockade in the reduction of antidepressant latency: personality variables and response to paroxetine and pindolol. J Affective Disord 44:101–109, 1997

Vedeniapin A, Anokhin A, Sirevaag, E, et al: P300 and personality in relation to personality disorders. Paper presented at the Psychophysiology Seminar, Department of Psychiatry, Washington University, St. Louis, MO, October 1997

Wilsson E, Sundgren PE: The use of a behaviour test for the selection of dogs for service and breeding, I: method of testing and evaluating test results in the adult dog, demands on different kinds of service dogs, sex and breed differences. Applied Animal Behaviour Science 53:279–295, 1997

Wodarz N, Wiesbeck GA, Rommelspacher H, et al: Excretion of beta-carbolines harman and norharman in 24-hour urine of chronic alcoholics during withdrawal and controlled abstinence. Alcohol Clin Exp Res 20:706–710, 1996

Chapter 4

Psychopharmacological Management of Personality Disorders: An Outcome-Focused Model

Paul S. Links, M.D., Ronald Heslegrave, Ph.D., and John Villella, M.Sc.

Our understanding of the biopsychosocial aspects of personality disorders is undergoing major alterations. The latest theoretical models are integrating genetic, biological, psychological, and social factors into the etiology and treatment of personality disorders while at the same time trying to clarify the unique contributions of each element (Paris 1996). With regards to biological research, Silk (1996) noted a major transition from focusing on the biological correlates of specific personality disorders to the more global approach of exploring underlying dimensions of personality variation. Ultimately these dimensions of personality are proposed to have specific ties to brain neurochemistry and neurophysiology. In light of these major revisions in our approach to the study of personality disorders, in this chapter we propose a new outcome-focused model for psychopharmacological management of personality disorders.

A number of reviewers of psychopharmacological research on personality disorders have struggled to clarify the role and purpose of pharmacological treatment in patients with personality disorders. Some authors have focused on the role of medication by examining specific drugs and drug types across a spectrum of disorders (Coccaro 1993; Soloff 1993). Other reviewers have commented on the efficacy of various drugs for a particular personality disorder diagnosis, such as borderline personality disorder (BPD) (Koenigsberg 1992; Links and Steiner 1988; Soloff 1993) or avoidant personality disorder (Deltito and Stam 1989). Recommendations for pharmacological interventions have been based on a purported understanding of the underlying biological mechanisms. For example, Soloff (1990) and Soloff et al. (1993) identified four areas of dyscontrol in borderline personality disorder to which pharmacotherapy could be targeted: 1) cognition, 2) affect, 3) impulse, and 4) anxiety. In a similar but slightly different approach, Silk (1996) suggested pursuing strategies based on dimensions of psychopathology rather than based on specific diagnoses. Gitlin (1993) outlined a strategy of pharmacotherapy based on the observed comorbidity between Axis I and II disorders. All of these dimensional approaches to the pharmacological treatment of personality disorders owe allegiance to the work of Siever and Davis (1991), who suggested that personality disorders could be best understood using a dimensional model grounded in the major Axis I syndromes. They proposed four dimensions of personality disorder psychopathology—cognitive perceptual, impulsivity and aggression, affective instability, and anxiety inhibition—dimensions that should guide the pharmacotherapy. Finally, Coccaro (1993) used a more empirical approach, suggesting that decisions regarding effective pharmacotherapy should be based on evidence from randomized, controlled trials.

In this chapter we begin with a discussion of some of the shortcomings of alternate approaches. The outcome-focused model is then discussed, highlighting the outcomes of specific behaviors, functioning and quality of life, the relationship between Axis I and II disorders, and outcomes based on psychobiological evidence. We conclude with some practical applications of adopting an outcome-focused approach to the psychopharmacological management of patients with personality disorders.

Shortcomings of Current Psychopharmacological Approaches

Koenigsberg (1992) outlined a number of different models to support the use of medication in patients with BPD. His structure serves as a useful framework to discuss some of the problems with alternate psychopharmacological approaches.

Biological Trait Model

The biological trait model considers personality disorders to have underlying biological temperaments, an assumption that is made throughout the chapters in this text. Temperament may be defined as a behavioral disposition that is present at birth (Rutter 1987), and purportedly temperament is more directly connected to neurobiological predispositions and vulnerabilities than to environmental experiences. Personality traits are known to have high heritability rates, usually in the range of 50% (Plomin 1990). Livesley et al. (1993) reported similar rates of heritability for 12 of 18 dimensions of personality disorders. However, the heritability of various personality traits is variable; for example, agreeableness is much less heritable than other broad dimensions of personality (Bergeman et al. 1993).

Although progress has been made in defining dimensions of personality, there remains debate as to the number of dimensions that are essential in a comprehensive theory of personality. For example, the five-factor model of personality (Costa and McCrae 1988) seems to define elements that may be close to temperament. The biological trait model attributes disordered personality to individuals being at the extremes of these defining dimensions (Paris 1996). However, the theoretical continuity between normal personality dimensions and personality disorders needs to be substantiated. This continuity model needs careful testing and would require large, randomly ascertained general population samples to be examined for personality disorder symptoms and examination of the distribution of these symptoms for such things as bimodality (Lenzenweger and Clarkin 1996). Discontinuities between personality disorder and normal personality may result from defining aspects of neurobiology such as the discontinuities that exist between some causes of mental retardation and normal IQ.

Tying underlying biological traits to the expression of clinical behaviors, affects, and cognitions is problematic. Affective instability serves as an example. The concept of affective instability may be understood based on Cloninger's concept of reward dependence (Cloninger 1987; Cloninger et al. 1993). Cloninger suggested that reward dependence may be related to a genetic dimension of personality and that the norepinephrine system may be responsible for modulating reward dependence. In this hypothesis, the heightened need for reward can leave the patient susceptible to rapid shifts in affective state. Other concepts of affective instability are more closely related to disinhibition of affect (van Reekum et al. 1994). The mechanism of disinhibition is more closely associated with the serotonergic system rather than the norepinephrine system. Although the biological trait model holds promise, considerable research has to be done before it has practical application to understanding clinical psychopathology and targeting pharmacological interventions.

Subsyndromal Model

The subsyndromal model, developed by Akiskal (1981), suggested that personality disorders are variants of Axis I disorders and not discrete diagnostic entities. BPD was considered a subsyndromal affective disorder, and attempts were made to seek biological markers that drew associations between Axis I and II disorders, such as depression and BPD (van Reekum et al. 1993). However, this area of study has now been exhausted because few promising leads were productive (van Reekum et al. 1993). With regard to BPD, Gunderson and Phillips (1991) critically reviewed the literature and concluded that the disorder was not simply an affective disorder. Although relationships between Axis I and II disorders exist, the subsyndromal model oversimplifies the nature of the associations. Siever and Davis (1991) provided a more elaborate model that categorized personality disorders based on a dimensional model grounded in Axis I syndromes.

Comorbidity or Diagnostically Focused Model

The diagnostically focused model suggests that the pharmacological treatment is driven by the specific diagnosis of the patient. That diagnosis may be an Axis II diagnosis or it may be a comorbid Axis II (found frequently) or Axis I (if any) diagnosis. This model is the most open to criticism. Gitlin (1993) pointed out a number of the methodological problems that exist with personality disorder diagnoses. First, the classification and nomenclature of Axis II disorders have gone through rapid shifts over the last two decades, leading to difficulties in providing a systematic body of research literature. There continue to be difficulties in establishing valid Axis II diagnoses. For example, very poor concordance exists between different structured interviews in making the same personality disorder diagnosis (Perry 1992). The validity of many of the categories of personality disorders remains in question (Paris 1996). Further, the field is frustrated by high rates of Axis II comorbidity. Evidence indicates that when one uses structured interviews (Nurnberg et al. 1991; Pfohl et al. 1986; Westen 1997), patients receiving one personality disorder diagnosis meet the criteria for several more concurrently. This lack of specificity makes it very difficult to attribute individual affective, cognitive, or behavioral characteristics to a particular disorder. Finally, each personality disorder has great heterogeneity within the disorder because individuals can meet the diagnostic criteria by evidencing different characteristics (Clarkin et al. 1983).

When comorbidity between Axis I and II disorders exists, several confounding effects may result when assessing a person's response to pharmacological treatment. An Axis I disorder affects a person's reporting of personality traits (Joffe and Regan 1988), and with resolution of the clinical disorder, the individual endorses less personality disturbance. In addition, Gitlin (1993) noted that when patients with comorbid disorders are treated with medication, it is difficult to ascertain the efficacy of the medication for the personality disorder itself versus the Axis I syndrome.

Symptom-Focused Model

The symptom-focused model suggests targeting pharmacotherapy based on specific symptoms. This model has some attractiveness because it would eschew any need for an etiologic understanding of personality disorders, and symptoms may provide measurable outcomes. However, several reviewers have noted that medications have very nonspecific effects when treating patients with personality disorders (Coccaro 1993; Links and Steiner 1988). For example, in patients with BPD, neuroleptic effectiveness is not restricted to improvement in psychotic-like symptoms but also impacts on anxiety, obsessive-compulsive symptoms, affective symptoms, and suicidal behavior (Gunderson and Links 1995). Studies of fluoxetine in patients with BPD have demonstrated improvement in depression, anxiety, paranoia, psychoticism, interpersonal sensitivity, obsessionality, hostility, and global functioning versus placebo comparisons (Gunderson and Links 1995; Soloff, in press). Koenigsberg (1992) questioned why medications typically have specific effects in particular Axis I disorders but are characterized by broad-spectrum effects in patients with BPD. This broad-spectrum action of medication may be related to several factors. Patients with BPD have high rates of placebo responsiveness (Soloff et al. 1993) that may lead to a global reporting of improvement. The lack of specificity of response may be related to measurement issues and the questionable reliability and validity of measures used to capture Axis II symptom patterns (Gitlin 1993).

Three examples of psychopathological features in which measurement issues must be addressed in order to foster further research are dissociative symptoms, affective lability, and impulsivity. Quasi-psychotic symptoms were added to the DSM-IV (American Psychiatric Association 1994) diagnostic criteria for BPD because clinical research supported their association with this diagnosis (Gunderson et al. 1991). Criterion nine in DSM-IV included transient, stress-related paranoid ideation and severe dissociative symptoms. Although advances have been made in the measurement of dissociative phenomena, are the dissociative aspects of an Axis II disturbance adequately captured by current instruments? For example, the Dissociative Experiences Scale (DES) was developed to quantify dissociative experience (Bernstein and Putman 1986). This scale is a self-report measure that assesses an individual's disturbances of identity, memory, awareness, depersonalization, derealization, and associated phenomena such as déjà vu or absorption. However, this scale does not assess the dissociation of moods or impulses so as not to overlap with psychopathology that may be more in the realm of affective disorders. These dissociative features, however, may be part of the severe dissociative symptoms that define BPD. The DES was found to have good test-retest reliability and adequate split-half reliability (Bernstein and Putman 1986). The validity of the DES for screening for dissociative experiences and disorders has been supported (Carlson et al. 1993; Steinberg et al. 1991). However, Norton et al. (1990) found that three subscales from the Symptom Checklist—90 (SCL—90) (Derogatis et al. 1974)—phobic anxiety, anger or hostility, and somatization—were predictive of the DES score. Dunn et al. (1993) found that an overall measure of psychological distress was quite predictive of DES scores in male veteran substance-abusing patients. Therefore, further study of the DES needs to account for the variance explained by anxiety symptoms, depression, and general psychopathology, particularly when used in samples of patients with Axis II disorders.

Affective lability, similarly, is a concept that requires further specification. As a personality trait, affective lability seems to be characterized by frequent, dramatic, and short-lasting mood swings within a 24-hour period. However, neuropsychiatrists use the concept of emotional lability to describe "emotional incontinence" found in patients with head injury, stroke, or multiple sclerosis (Iannaccone and Ferini-Strambi 1996). Are these concepts related? Is variation in mood different from mixed mood states? The Visual Analogue Mood Scale (VAMS) has been used to measure mood stability and instability and has documented psychometric characteristics (Folstein and Luria 1973). Subjects rate their mood multiple times a day over several days and record the rating on a continuous 100-mm straight line anchored by descriptors at either end (i.e., "worst I've ever felt" and "best I've ever felt") (Cowdry et al. 1991). The VAMS method requires compliance with multiple testing sessions, and thus must be very simple and nonintrusive. Concerns have also been raised that the multiple retesting may lead to regression toward the mean (Little and Penman 1989). The Affective Lability Scale (ALS) has also been purported as a measure of affective lability (Harvey et al. 1989). The ALS is a self-report measure of changeable affect, and the subject cross-sectionally completes questions related to changes in affect from euthymia to depression, anxiety, anger, and hypomania and shifts from hypomania and depression and anxiety and depression (Harvey et al. 1989). However, ALS has not been adequately studied in clinical populations. The General Behavior Inventory (GBI) is a reliable and valid instrument developed to assess current cyclothymia including biphasic symptoms (Depue et al. 1981). Our group is presently trying to determine the concordance between various measures of affective lability including the VAMS, ALS, and GBI in an adult inpatient sample. Clarification of these measurement issues must proceed so that psychopharmacological intervention trials will have adequate outcome measures to incorporate into future studies.

Impulsivity is a widely used concept but the term is employed to characterize a variety of psychopathological features. Neuropsychologists speak of rapid, poorly planned test taking responses, psychiatrists may focus on overt behaviors such as reckless driving or self-harm behaviors, and pediatricians may focus on inattention and motor restlessness (van Reekum et al. 1994). Progress is being made to relate measures of impulsivity to underlying neurobiological mechanisms, which will be discussed in more detail in the next section.

Summary of Alternative Approaches

Ultimately each of these four approaches to the psychopharmacological management of personality disorders has merit. The clinician can develop a rationale for psychopharmacological management of personality disorders based on these approaches, and Soloff's symptom-specific classification for psychopharmacological management is the most well developed. Soloff (in press) has recently presented a treatment algorithm based on evidence for efficacy, safety, and rapidity of action of particular treatments. Gunderson and Links (1995) have used a similar organization to familiarize clinicians with the role of medications in BPD. Using this organization, the medication of first choice can be determined. For example, for cognitive-perceptual disturbances including dissociative symptoms, low-dose neuroleptics are the medication of first choice, based on efficacy, safety, and rapidity of response (Soloff, in press). Selective serotonin reuptake inhibitors (SSRIs) such as fluoxetine are the first-line treatment for affective dysregulation or dyscontrol. The second-line approach for affective symptoms is the use of monoamine oxidase inhibitors (MAOIs); this finding is based on two randomized, controlled trials (Cowdry and Gardner 1988; Soloff et al. 1993). Tricyclic antidepressants have not been shown to be effective for affective symptoms, particularly in patients with BPD (Links et al. 1990b; Soloff et al. 1986). Despite much discussion, the role of mood stabilizers in regulating affect in BPD has not been well supported for lithium, carbamazepine, or valproate (de la Fuente and Lotstra 1994; Links et al. 1990b; Stein et al. 1995), though there are a few open studies that suggest that valproic acid may be useful in patients with BPD (Stein et al. 1995; Wilcox 1995). If impulsive behavior is the target symptom, evidence suggests that SSRIs such as fluoxetine are the agents of choice. Antianxiety agents are thought to play little role in the treatment of Axis II disorders because of the potential for abuse, reported disinhibition that can lead to increased impulsivity (Cowdry and Gardner 1988), and long delay before effectiveness is demonstrated, particularly with buspirone.

Although the symptom-specific approach has merit in terms of providing a rationale for psychopharmacological management, we believe it also has inherent dangers. During the past decade, the use of medication, specifically for BPD patients, has changed from being an occasional intervention to an expected one. Such thinking may then foster the use of medication without adequate scientific justification. We suggest that while the neurochemical and neurobiological substrates of underlying dimensions of the personality disorders are being clarified, attention should turn to the outcome sought from psychopharmacological management of patients with personality disorders. The focus on specific outcomes will allow psychopharmacologists to target interventions more effectively, to measure the effects of this intervention more precisely, and, in turn, to facilitate our understanding of the psychobiological mechanisms supporting these outcomes.

Outcome-Focused Model

The rationale for an outcome-focused model is to 1) clearly delineate the purpose of a psychopharmacological intervention for both the patient and clinician, 2) choose outcomes that are measurable and related to functional improvements, and 3) further our understanding of the underlying psychobiological mechanisms. Finally, an outcome-focused approach may make the development of new psychopharmacological approaches for patients with personality disorders of more relevance and interest to funding agencies and drug manufacturers. The following suggests specific outcomes that should be targeted using an outcome-focused approach.

Specific Behaviors

Specific behaviors provide definable and measurable outcomes even when the underlying neurobiological mechanisms are not well understood. Demonstrating the effectiveness of an intervention can then lead to a subsequent clarification of the mechanisms involved. Some examples of specific behaviors for psychopharmacological investigation include self-harm behaviors, suicidal behaviors, treatment adherence, and individual patient-specific outcomes.

Self-Harm Behavior

Self-harm behavior is a disturbing but challenging behavior that is particularly characteristic of BPD. This observable and documentable behavior tends to be resistant to treatment (Roth et al. 1996) but also characterizes a group of BPD patients who demonstrate twice the risk of suicide compared with patients without self-injurious behavior (Linehan et al. 1991). Self-harm behavior is poorly characterized (Winchel and Stanley 1991) and can have a number of attributes; for example, self-harm behavior may or may not have accompanying suicidal intent, may be associated with a sense of emotional relief, may be accompanied by an analgesic response to tissue damage, and in some cases may lead to sexual arousal. Although refinement of this concept is required, self-harm behavior still provides an opportunity for very measurable outcomes. In addition, some promising biological models have been developed to explain self-harm behavior and to offer opportunities for intervention.

Self-harm behavior may be related to a dysregulation of the endorphin neurotransmitter system (Winchel and Stanley 1991) and is frequently associated with childhood histories of traumatic abuse and neglect (Links et al. 1990a). Childhood abuse is hypothesized to lead to endorphin system dysfunction and ultimately to self-mutilation (van der Kolk 1996). The self-harm behavior may be perpetuated because of the reinforcing properties of endogenous opioids that are released during the injurious behavior (Lienemann and Walker 1989; Winchel and Stanley 1991).

A common mechanism is proposed for a number of characteristics of BPD. These characteristics—self-mutilation, binge eating, flashbacks, and substance abuse—may all be perpetuated by a release of increased endogenous opioids that reinforces the problematic behavior. Binge eating is an impulsive behavior found in patients with BPD. Bulimic women have been found to have lower plasma β-endorphin concentration than controls (Waller et al. 1986) and lower cerebrospinal fluid (CSF) concentrations of β-endorphins then controls (Brewerton et al. 1992). Recurrent flashbacks to traumatic experiences have been related to endogenous opioids (Bills and Kreisler 1993). Naltrexone is an opioid receptor antagonist felt to have potential to prevent the reinforcing effects of endogenous opioid release and thus can act to decrease the repetitive behaviors outlined.

The enthusiasm for using naltrexone in self-harm behavior comes from several lines of evidence. Self-harm behavior has been a focus of interventions with individuals with mental retardation. Willemsen-Swinkels et al. (1995) reviewed the evidence and indicated that a decrease in self-harm behavior was found in about 70% of patients treated with naloxone (short-acting antagonist) and naltrexone (long-acting antagonist); however, most reports had been pilot studies using small numbers of subjects or uncontrolled designs. These authors completed a randomized, controlled trial involving mentally retarded autistic adults and compared active treatment with naltrexone (either 50 mg/day or 150 mg/day) versus placebo. Their study found that naltrexone was not effective in decreasing self-harm behavior and in fact increased incidents of stereotypic behavior. The findings were taken as not supportive of the use of naltrexone in mentally retarded autistic adults.

The usefulness of naltrexone in patients with BPD comes from case reports. Roth et al. (1996) published a report of seven females with self-harm behavior who had been particularly refractory to other treatments. Each of the patients had self-harm behavior accompanied by analgesia and a reduction in dysphoria. In an open-label design, all patients received 50 mg/day of naltrexone with a mean follow-up period of 10.7 weeks. The study is interesting because the patients were found to have marked responses to the naltrexone, with a total elimination of self-harm behavior in six out of the seven patients. In two patients, there was a rapid recurrence of self-harm behavior when the naltrexone treatment was interrupted, but when the medication was reinstituted the behaviors stopped. The authors suggested that naltrexone was particularly useful for individuals who have self-harm behavior accompanied by analgesia and dysphoric reduction. In another case report by McGee (1997), the treatment of a female patient with BPD and persistent self-harm behavior was discussed. The patient, after many treatment failures, received naltrexone (50 mg/day), which was effective in helping the patient maintain sobriety and dramatically diminished her self-harm behavior. The report is interesting for two reasons: 1) it demonstrates that again naltrexone has dramatic effects on self-harm behavior and 2) it hints at an interactive effect between the reduction of alcohol abuse and the elimination of self-harm behavior.

Naltrexone is of particular interest with BPD because of the high comorbidity with alcohol abuse. Links et al. (1988) found that in a sample of inpatients with BPD, approximately 30% met lifetime criteria for the diagnosis of alcoholism. In our own follow-up sample of BPD patients, individuals initially diagnosed with BPD and substance abuse reported more evidence of impulsive behaviors, suicide attempts, and self-mutilation on follow-up compared with patients with BPD without concurrent substance abuse (Links et al. 1995). The demonstrated effectiveness of naltrexone in maintaining abstinence from alcohol may have benefits with substance-abusing, self-mutilative patients.

With regard to alcohol abstinence, Volpicelli et al. (1992) completed a randomized, controlled trial of 70 male alcoholic patients drawn mainly from a veterans' health center. The patients were randomized to receive naltrexone (50 mg/day) or placebo as an adjunct to outpatient alcohol treatment. During the 12-week study, only 23% of the naltrexone-treated subjects met criteria for relapse versus 54.3% of the placebo-treated subjects. Naltrexone was particularly effective in patients who had a slip toward reinitiating drinking during their outpatient treatment. Of the 20 placebo-treated patients, 19 (95%) relapsed after sampling alcohol, while only 8 of 16 (50%) patients treated with naltrexone suffered an alcohol relapse.

The second major study was carried out by O'Malley et al. (1992), who demonstrated the effectiveness of naltrexone in 97 alcohol-dependent patients. The sample consisted primarily of white males, with an average age of 40 years. The study had four conditions: naltrexone (50 mg/day) plus psychotherapy that was either a supportive psychotherapy module (mainly to encourage the patient to remain abstinent) or coping skills relapse prevention therapy versus placebo plus either of the psychotherapy modules. With regard to the outcome of abstinence, 61% of the naltrexone supportive therapy group abstained continuously over the 12 weeks of follow-up, whereas the rates of continuous abstinence were 28% for the subjects in the naltrexone/coping skills group, 21% for the subjects in the placebo/coping skills group, and 19% for the subjects in the placebo/supportive group. Similar to the Volpicelli et al. (1992) study, O'Malley reported that naltrexone decreased the risk of heavy drinking after the first slip. Patients taking naltrexone reported decreased craving for alcohol, which is hypothesized as the mechanism preventing the slip from becoming a full relapse. This evidence suggests that naltrexone may be particularly useful in decreasing the reinforcing effects of the first alcoholic drink, thereby preventing a trial of drinking from leading to a full relapse.

Given the promising evidence for naltrexone in decreasing self-harm behavior and alcohol abuse, we are proposing a randomized, controlled trial using naltrexone versus placebo in patients with BPD and determining the effectiveness on a number of repetitive behaviors including self-harm. The patients will be stratified based on the presence or absence of alcohol abuse.

Repetitive Suicidal Behavior

Repetitive suicidal behavior provides a specific outcome for psychopharmacological trials. Repeated suicide attempts and threats are characteristic of patients with BPD and identify a group at high risk for completed suicide (Links et al. 1996). Some evidence points to pharmacological interventions as having a role in decreasing the risk of suicidal behaviors in patients with a repetitive pattern of such behavior.

Montgomery and Montgomery (1982) carried out a study using low-dose flupentixol (20 mg every 4 weeks) compared with placebo. Patients were admitted to the hospital with a suicide attempt and were screened for schizophrenic, depressive, or organic illness. The patients had to have a history of two or more documented suicide attempts and then were randomized to receive either active medication or placebo. The sample included patients with personality disorders, most commonly with borderline or histrionic features. The patients were followed for 6 months. Compared with placebo, the flupentixol group showed a significant reduction in the number of suicidal acts at 4 and 5 months' follow-up, and this difference continued to be highly significant at 6 months' follow-up. Montgomery and Montgomery indicated that "this was the first report of a positive effect of pharmacotherapy or indeed any treatment in reducing subsequent suicidal acts in patients prone to suicidal behavior" (p. 295).

The other line of evidence suggesting antisuicidal properties from medication comes from experience with lithium-treated bipolar affective disorder patients (Schou 1997). Schou, in reviewing the effectiveness of lithium on mortality in patients given long-term lithium treatment, notes that the mortality rate, in general, for manic-depressive patients is markedly higher than for the general population and that this increased rate is mainly a result of suicide. A series of mortality studies conducted on long-term lithium-treated patients indicated that the mortality of these patients is markedly lower than patients at risk who have not received lithium treatment. Using the International Group for the Study of Lithium-Treated Patients, which collected data on 5,600 patient years, the standardized mortality ratios for patients on long-term lithium were not significantly higher than in the general population. A second observation comes from patients who were started on lithium but then were noncompliant. These patients have mortality and suicide rates significantly higher than the general population. Lastly, Schou reports on advantages of lithium to prevent suicidal behavior based on a particular multicenter trial. Patients have been randomized to receive lithium or carbamazepine for bipolar illness or treatment with lithium or amitriptyline for unipolar illness. Among the patients taking antidepressant drugs, there were five suicides and no suicide attempts; for carbamazepine, there were four suicides and four suicide attempts; in the lithium-treated group, there were no suicides and no suicide attempts. Schou presents the hypothesis that lithium treatment in these patient groups actually protects against suicidal behavior.

This hypothesis is of interest because of a preliminary report on a double-blind, random-order placebo crossover trial of lithium and desipramine versus placebo in patients with BPD. Unfortunately, the study was characterized by a high dropout rate, and only 58.8% of patients were able to complete two or more arms of the study (Links et al. 1990b). However, the study showed a trend for decreased reports of anger and suicidal symptoms in patients taking lithium versus desipramine. While taking lithium, 8 of 11 patients showed a response (72.2%) versus 4 of 11 patients taking desipramine (36.4%) ($P = .09$). The therapist also rated lithium as significantly superior to placebo, and there was a trend for lithium to be rated superior to desipramine. The therapist seemed to be identifying a positive response based on a decrease in the patients' irritability, anger, and evidence of suicidal symptoms (Links et al. 1990b).

SSRIs may prevent suicidal behavior by affecting the regulation of the serotonergic system and thereby decreasing aggression and irritability (Coccaro et al. 1989). Reviewing previous trials, SSRIs were found to be effective for reducing hostility, impulsiveness, and self-destructive or suicidal behavior (Gunderson and Links 1995). Some of the evidence comes from Markowitz and colleagues' (1991) study, which demonstrated a decrease in self-injurious suicidal behavior after treatment with fluoxetine, and the study by Kavoussi et al. (1994), which demonstrated significant reductions in overt aggression and irritability in patients treated with sertraline in an open, pre- to post-treatment comparison. The SSRIs, typically, were effective for a wide range of symptoms; however, the changes in impulsivity and hostility were seen as independent of any effect on depressive symptoms.

Specific intervention trials should be developed to determine whether these or other medications that regulate the serotonergic system will reduce the risk of repetitive suicidal behavior in individuals at high risk for recurrent suicidal behavior. Researchers have missed opportunities to study this outcome along with other outcomes in individuals at high risk for suicidal behavior (i.e., by studying medications to prevent relapse in alcoholic subjects but not recording the impact of suicidal behaviors). Through targeted pharmacological investigations, the biological mechanisms leading to suicidal behavior may be further understood.

Treatment Adherence

A focused outcome relevant for patients with personality disorders is their compliance or adherence to treatment. This variable is important to such patients for several reasons. First, patients with personality disorders, specifically BPD, fail to complete treatment in high numbers. A prospective study of 60 young adult BPD inpatients referred for psychotherapy and pharmacotherapy indicated that 43% of patients failed to complete 6 months of treatment (Gunderson et al. 1989). Similar high dropout rates occur in pharmacological studies, including our study, where approximately 40% of the sample dropped out, greatly limiting the generalizability of the findings (Links et al. 1990b). Cowdry and Gardner (1988) found that only 50%–60% of their sample went through to completion during their pharmacotherapy study.

Adherence is recognized by both clinicians and empirical investigators to be related to the clinical outcome. Kernberg (1975) considered threats to continuity of treatment as one of the highest priorities when working with patients with BPD. Waldinger and Gunderson (1984) suggested that the efficacy of specific treatments for BPD proved to be more effective the longer patients remained in treatment. The psychotherapy literature suggests that individuals with personality disorders require increased length of treatment versus other disorders for the treatment to be effective in making changes. The relationship between length of psychotherapy treatment and symptom improvement has been effectively shown by Howard and colleagues (1986) and Kopta and colleagues (1994). Both their earlier and later reports indicated that individuals with personality disorders require up to 52 sessions of individual therapy in order that 50% of patients will show recovery. Linehan's (1991) study of patients with parasuicidal BPD was one of the few trials to demonstrate effectiveness, and increased treatment adherence differentiated the active treatment group compared with the treatment-as-usual group. Individuals in the intervention group had a 100% maintenance rate versus the 73% retention rate in the treatment-as-usual group. Given that interventions for patients with personality disorders are likely to be multimodal, psychopharmacological interventions are often combined with psychotherapeutic techniques. Patients' outcomes are affected by their adherence to the total treatment regimen. Monitoring the adherence to both the medication and the psychotherapeutic intervention is an important component of outcome.

The continuity of treatment appears to be achieved when patients' anger and hostility are addressed. Kelly et al. (1992) indicated that more effective strategies for "managing the borderline patients' anger and impulsiveness early in the treatment are necessary to protect the course of therapy" (p. 429). In this study, they found that individuals who failed to complete treatment were more behaviorally impulsive and overtly hostile than the more compliant individuals. Similarly, Gunderson et al. (1989) found that therapeutic confrontation activated BPD patients' anger toward the therapist and was the cause of patients dropping out early. Interventions targeted at decreasing anger and impulsivity and improving adherence to treatment may be associated with the best overall outcomes. As indicated, the impulsivity may be affected by employing SSRIs, and adherence to the overall treatment plan should be measured as an important outcome.

Patient-Specific Outcomes

Choosing patient-specific outcomes can be important when working with patients with personality disorders. This suggestion relates to a number of difficulties inherent in treating patients with personality disorders. Patients within the same diagnostic category often can be heterogeneous and therefore may be characterized by very individualized responses to medication. Coccaro (1993) identified that even within a carefully designed study, the therapeutic effects of different agents within the same patient were not correlated with each other. For example, Cowdry and Gardner (1988) reported that the correlation and global ratings of response between carbamazepine and tranylcypromine within patients were approaching zero. Even in carefully conceived studies, there seems to be little correlation between

---

self-reported outcomes and observer-rated outcomes as documented by both Links et al. (1990b) and Soloff et al. (1986).

Given the preceding considerations, the psychopharmacologist should target the intervention trial of a specific patient to patient-specific outcomes. An N of 1 trial design may be used to test the value of a particular medication regime compared with previous therapy in a patient with a personality disorder. This methodology seems useful to engage the patient in therapy and to encourage him or her to carefully define the priority outcomes for himself or herself. This approach appears to have particular merit for patients with borderline and other personality disorders because it encourages their collaboration in assessing the medication and diminishes their fears of being controlled externally, preventing a long-term commitment to medication that may do more harm than good and making expectations for outcome of the medication clearer. In developing an N of 1 study, the details of setting up a within-patient randomized trial can be reviewed in Guyatt et al. (1988). The patient should be an active participant, work to identify the specific outcomes, and develop means for monitoring these outcomes over time. As part of the preparation, the clinician should assess the patient for symptoms, particularly symptoms that might be consistent with the side effect profile of medication, before starting the medication. This evaluation provides a baseline for monitoring the appearance of new symptoms during the trial of medications and also provides a better baseline by which to judge the emergence and prevalence of side effects. We have published the results of an N of 1 trial, looking at the use of methylphenidate in a female patient with BPD and childhood history of attention-deficit/hyperactivity disorder (van Reekum and Links 1994).

Functional Outcomes and Quality of Life

Future psychopharmacological trials in patients with personality disorders should be focused on functional outcomes. Little research has been undertaken to provide correlations between diagnoses of personality disorders, symptom status, and performance in social roles. Certain diagnostic categories of personality disorders tend to be associated with lower levels of functioning (Nakao et al. 1992). However, functional status seems to vary markedly among patients with personality disorders and even within different social contexts for the same patient. Results of previous long-term follow-up studies suggested that BPD patients are characterized as being less dysfunctional in work roles than they appear to be in social, leisure, and family roles (McGlashan 1985; Paris et al. 1987; Stone 1990). We provided some evidence that symptom status was related to role performance and found affective and impulsive symptoms inversely related to good social role performance in a sample of BPD patients assessed 2 years after an inpatient admission (Links 1993). Paris (1996) maintained that pretreatment functional levels may be very useful in deciding on patients' treatability and targeting patients for particular treatments. Overall, functional status may assist with treatment assignment and assessment of treatment outcome and therefore requires further study.

In considering the outcome-focused approach to delineate the efficacy of pharmacological interventions with patients with personality disorders, one functional and measurable outcome that has received little attention in psychiatry until recently and virtually no attention in the personality disorders literature is the quality of life (QOL) of affected patients. A literature search for the past 2 years of MEDLINE failed to reveal any articles that measured QOL in patients with personality disorders, though QOL is measured in other psychiatric disorders including anxiety (Sherbourne et al. 1996) and panic disorders (Hollifield et al. 1997).

QOL has been used as an evaluative tool in medicine for many years but has only recently been applied in psychiatry (Lehman 1983; Lehman et al. 1982, 1986). For example, there has recently been a great deal of interest in evaluating the QOL of patients with schizophrenia (Awad 1992). Of more specific interest to this chapter, however, is that in the last few years QOL has been suggested as an evaluative tool with respect to psychopharmacological interventions (Awad et al. 1997). In terms of Axis II disorders, QOL measures have received little or no attention, yet patients with personality disorders commonly report, and are characterized by, symptoms that would impact on the various dimensions subsumed under the QOL concept. By evaluating QOL in patients with personality disorders, it may be possible to bring new evidence and understanding to the role and value of psychopharmacology in the treatment of personality disorders that extends beyond the control of symptoms. In this sense, QOL indicators can help to balance the impact of pharmacological treatment focused on symptom reduction with functional improvement by providing patient-oriented, subjectively based, and objectively measured assessments of both symptom and functional improvement. However, since studies in QOL are largely absent from the personality disorders literature, conceptual and empirical lessons learned from other areas of application within psychiatry should be used as guideposts for the development of QOL measures that can be applied to the study of personality disorders.

QOL has been defined in many ways that have been both vague and better defined. Conceptually, QOL has been viewed as a broad concept incorporating dimensions such as health, employment, family, environment, social relations, and goals and aspirations. However, the breadth of the concept can make its measurement difficult. For this and other reasons, various refinements have been made in the definition of QOL. Perhaps the most important refinement has been to restrict QOL to health-related QOL in terms of its application to chronic diseases. As prolonged life expectancy through more efficacious treatment has turned many life-threatening diseases into chronic diseases, including cardiovascular disease, cancer, and schizophrenia, disease-related debilitation or reduced health-related QOL has become more of a focus for QOL research since it targets the limiting factors related to the specific diseases and treatments. In terms of psychiatry, the recent conceptualizations in defining health-related QOL for schizophrenia would be a useful starting point in terms of defining an approach to the QOL issues in personality disorders.

In a recent approach to the study of QOL in schizophrenia,

Awad (1992) and Awad and colleagues (1997) have developed a conceptual model to define QOL in patients with schizophrenia who are maintained on antipsychotic pharmacological therapy. This conceptual model of QOL for schizophrenia (Awad 1992) proposes that the health-related QOL for chronic schizophrenic patients maintained on antipsychotic medication is largely a function of symptoms, side effects, and psychosocial performance. Moreover, the severity of psychotic symptoms, the subjective and objective responses to medication, and the level and quality of psychosocial interaction account for a significant degree of the variation in the QOL reported by schizophrenic patients. Although other factors such as premorbid adjustment, resources, social networks, attitudes, education, and personality characteristics inevitably play a modulating role in these patients, it has been proposed that the primary factors of symptoms, medication side effects, and psychosocial interactions are the primary determinants of changes in QOL. As a preliminary test of this new conceptual model, Awad and colleagues (1997) used the Sickness Impact Profile (Bergner et al. 1981) to assess QOL; the Positive and Negative Symptom Scale (Kay et al. 1989) to assess symptoms; the Hillside Akathisia Scale (Fleishhacker et al. 1989), Abnormal Involuntary Movement Scale (Department of Health, Education, and Welfare), and Drug Attitude Inventory (Hogan et al. 1983) to assess objective and subjective side effects of medication; and the Social Performance Schedule and Global Scale of Adaptive Functioning (Axis V) to assess psychosocial functioning. This study showed that almost half of the variance in QOL scores could be accounted for by the severity of symptoms (32%) and the subjective distress caused by akathisia (11%) and neuroleptic dysphoria (6%). Given this relatively strong initial confirmation of a conceptual model (though psychosocial functioning was not a strong, independent predictor of QOL using this specific QOL measure), perhaps a similar approach should be adopted to study the impact of personality disorders and pharmacological treatment for such disorders on the QOL of patients with personality disorders.

In summary, QOL has recently been applied in psychiatry, with interesting results. More importantly, it is a method of describing the current functional status of patients with personality disorders that incorporates their symptoms, side effects, and current functional status. If one is going to take a psychopharmacological approach to the treatment of personality disorders, then appropriate QOL measures need to be developed to assess the impact of the psychiatric, psychological, and pharmacological interventions on these patients in a balanced fashion.

Treatment Based on Association or Relationship to Axis I Disorders

A strategy that should take the highest priority with Axis II patients is the treatment of definitive comorbid Axis I disorders (Links and Steiner 1988; Soloff 1993). Gitlin (1993) argued that this strategy was most important when the personality disorder is "reminiscent constitutionally" of the Axis I disorder. If there is conceptual overlap between the criteria for the Axis I and II disorders, or if the disorders are related based on biological mechanisms, then targeting the Axis I disorder provides a very realistic focus for psychopharmacological management of patients with personality disorders.

Targeting an Axis I disorder to modify an Axis II disorder is best demonstrated by considering avoidant personality disorder. Avoidant personality disorder is a relatively new category in DSM-IV and characterizes patients with long-standing, pervasive, and active withdrawal from social relationships (Deltito and Stam 1989). Avoidant personality disorder overlaps considerably with the concept of generalized or global social phobia. Generalized or global social phobia relates to patients who exhibit a generalized fear of social situations such as speaking to strangers or going out in social situations (Deltito and Stam 1989). Liebowitz et al. (1992) argued that there may be important differences in pharmacological response between generalized and discrete social phobia. Evidence from a number of trials indicates that as social phobic symptoms improved, the number of avoidant personality traits was reduced. Reich et al. (1989) examined whether alprazolam affected avoidant personality traits in 14 patients with social phobia. First, the authors demonstrated considerable overlap between social phobia and cluster C Axis II disorders. Second, alprazolam significantly reduced many avoidant personality symptoms, and these symptoms correlated highly with reductions in measures of anxiety and functional disability. Liebowitz et al. (1992) focused on generalized social phobia and were able to demonstrate that phenelzine was significantly superior to placebo and atenolol. This finding supported their proposal that generalized social phobia is more akin to avoidant personality disorder than to discrete social phobia. Liebowitz and colleagues likened the response in generalized social phobia to the efficacy that has been found in atypical depression. Changes in interpersonal hypersensitivity occurred with phenelzine in atypical depression and may explain the response in patients with avoidant personality disorder. Liebowitz et al. concluded that their "data suggests that avoidant personality features in patients with social phobias are phenelzine responsive" (p. 299). Versiani et al. (1992) demonstrated that moclobemide and phenelzine were more effective than placebo in changing the number of avoidant criteria met by patients with social phobia. By 8 weeks of treatment, only three patients taking the active drug still met criteria for avoidant personality disorder, with 14 of 16 of the placebo group still fulfilling criteria (Versiani et al. 1992). Fahlen (1995) found that the maladaptive personality traits characteristic of social phobias that included avoidant traits were very responsive to brofaromine. The authors demonstrated that the number of patients meeting criteria for avoidant personality disorder had diminished from 60% at the beginning of the trial to 20% at completion. Van Ameringen and colleagues (1993, 1994) studied the effectiveness of SSRIs in the treatment of generalized social phobia. They showed that measures of social anxiety and phobia avoidance were significantly improved pre- to posttreatment with fluoxetine or sertraline. As of yet, the study of SSRIs in patients with social phobia has not focused on changes in Axis II psychopathology.

Social phobia and avoidant personality disorder demonstrate that when Axis I and II disorders are conceptually or biologically related, targeting an Axis I disorder for treatment impacts the

Axis II disorder. A similar relationship might be proposed in targeting social withdrawal or the negative symptoms of schizotypal personality disorder for intervention. In general, the use of low-dose neuroleptics has led to benefits not restricted to the psychotic-like symptoms. Novel antipsychotics might be used to target the social withdrawal or negative features of schizotypal personality disorder, paralleling some success reported in the negative symptoms of schizophrenia. Depression in patients with personality disorders is often the target of psychopharmacological intervention. The nature of the relationship between clinical depression and Axis II disorders is probably multidetermined, partly an artifact of the overlapping clinical features and partly because of shared vulnerability related to biological, psychological, and social issues. The comorbid personality disorder affects the treatment response of depression to medication. The treatment response tends to be poorer in comorbid patients (Links 1996); however, with resolution of the acute episode of depression, comorbid patients endorse less personality dysfunction, as shown by changes in self-report measures of personality dysfunction (Joffe and Regan 1988). By carefully characterizing the relationship between Axis I and II disorders, we may be better able to target pharmacological interventions. With our current knowledge, in many cases, appropriate pharmacological treatment of the Axis I disorder will lead to resolution of some of the Axis II psychopathology.

Outcomes Based on Psychobiological Data

For the future, tying outcomes more closely to the psychobiological dimensions of personality and personality disorders is of particular importance. Coccaro (1993) provided a step-by-step approach to the establishment of how a specific biological dimension may be a target of psychopharmacological therapy. First, Coccaro et al. (1989) built on other biological data by showing that a pharmacological challenge test, in this case fenfluramine challenge, was highly correlated with measures of irritability and aggression, regardless of diagnosis. Coccaro and colleagues' next step was to seek a specific outcome measure capable of assessing behaviors that were mediated by this central serotonergic activity. The authors used their data from the prolactin response to fenfluramine to develop both a self-report and clinician-rated assessment of impulsive aggression (Coccaro et al. 1991). They then undertook the third step of testing the value of specific and selective serotonergic agents such as sertraline in patients characterized by impulsive aggressiveness. Kavoussi et al. (1994) completed an open trial in 11 patients who were characterized as having impulsive aggressiveness. The results indicated that 9 of the 11 patients completed at least 4 weeks of treatment and showed significant changes in overt aggression and irritability levels. The changes in overt aggression seemed to predate improvement in irritability, and this improvement required patients to participate in the trial for at least 4 weeks. The authors found no significant correlation between measures of anxiety and depression and measures of aggression or irritability at baseline or termination of the study. Coccaro et al. (1997) have recently confirmed these findings with a randomized controlled trial that demonstrated the effectiveness of fluoxetine for personality disordered patients with impulsive aggressiveness. This example provides a model for developing very specific outcomes to target based on specific dimensions of personality disorder and their association with neurobiological findings. Although Coccaro and colleagues should be recognized for their careful step-by-step approach, many questions remain to be answered. For example, it is not clear whether their results would be applicable to female subjects. Coccaro et al. (1991) emphasized behavioral irritability based on their sample. Van Reekum et al. (1994) studied a group of patients with BPD that included a preponderance of females. In this sample, anger and a predisposition to feeling "ready to explode" characterized the subjects' impulsivity. Female subjects may not be impulsive interpersonally but rather self-direct impulsivity, resulting in increased suicidality (van Reekum et al. 1994). Overall, Coccaro's demonstration of a step-by-step approach to characterizing the psychopathological outcomes that connect to psychobiological hypotheses and data provides a model on which future investigators may build.

Conclusions

The approach outlined in this chapter provides some guidance for clinicians:

1. Attempts to target pharmacological therapy based on proposed biological dimensions or symptom patterns are not well established. Although research in this area should be supported, it requires a very careful step-by-step approach, as discussed previously.
2. Focusing pharmacological management against a specific Axis II diagnosis is not supported.
3. Axis I disorders in patients with Axis I and II comorbidity should receive high priority for psychopharmacological management. The comorbid Axis II disorder may be an additional target of therapy in patients when it is conceptually or biologically reminiscent of the Axis I disorder in question.
4. Particular behavioral targets seem to be rational outcomes for a focus of pharmacological interventions. As discussed earlier, self-harm, repetitive suicidal behavior, treatment adherence, and specific patient-defined behaviors are appropriate for pharmacological trials. These examples provide an opportunity to develop meaningful outcomes and eventually to test specific biological hypotheses, such as the importance of endogenous opioids in the perpetuation of self-harm behavior.
5. Pharmacological interventions may well be used to facilitate the patient's availability for other therapy approaches. In a crisis situation, medications may be used to dampen a broad spectrum of symptoms (Links and Steiner 1988). In the longer term, trying to improve adherence to other therapies through psychopharmacological treatment can be monitored as an important outcome. Facilitating adherence likely

makes the patient more available for other modalities of therapy and has a meaningful impact on the overall outcome.

6. Patient-specific outcomes are encouraged. An *N* of 1 design is a useful strategy to employ with a particular patient and an effective way to actively involve the patient in the pharmacological procedure.

7. Pharmacological management should be directed at improving patient functioning. An important outcome of a pharmacological trial is improved functioning including work, family, and other aspects of social role performance. In the future, QOL indicators may also be used to measure the effectiveness of pharmacological interventions and provide a better assessment of the balance between symptom reduction, side effects, and functioning in various QOL dimensions.

In conclusion, the future may well hold the possibility of targeting pharmacological interventions at specific psychobiological dimensions of personality disorders. However, this approach requires an extensive body of research to make meaningful connections between these dimensions and clinical outcomes. In the meantime, pharmacological trials can be focused on various aspects of outcome, and we have highlighted an approach focused on aspects of outcome including behaviors, function, QOL, and the relationships to Axis I disorders.

References

Akiskal HS: Subaffective disorders: dysthymic, cyclothymic, and bipolar II disorders in the "borderline" realm. Psychiatr Clin North Am 4:25–46, 1981

American Psychiatric Association: Diagnostic and Statistical Manual of Mental Disorders, 4th Edition. Washington, DC, American Psychiatric Association, 1994

Awad AG: Quality of life of schizophrenic patients on medications and implications for new drug trials. Hosp Comm Psychiatry 43:262–265, 1992

Awad AG, Voruganti NLP, Heslegrave RJ: A conceptual model of quality of life in schizophrenia: description and preliminary clinical validation. Qual Life Res 6:21–26, 1997

Bergeman CS, Chipeur HM, Plomin R, et al: Genetic and environmental effects on openness to experience, agreeableness, and conscientiousness: an adoption/twin study. J Pers 61:158–179, 1993

Bergner M, Bobbit RA, Carter WB, et al: The Sickness Impact Profile: reliability of a health status measure. Med Care 19:787–805, 1981

Bernstein EM, Putman FW: Development, reliability, and validity of a dissociation scale. J Nerv Ment Dis 174:727–735, 1986

Bills LJ, Kreisler K: Treatment of flashbacks with naltrexone (letter). Am J Psychiatry 150:1430, 1993

Brewerton TD, Lydiard RB, Laraia MT, et al: CSF β-endorphin and dynorphin in bulimia nervosa. Am J Psychiatry 149:1086–1090, 1992

Carlson EB, Putman FW, Ross CA, et al: Validity of the Dissociative Experiences Scale in screening for multiple personality disorder: a multicenter study. Am J Psychiatry 150:1030–1036, 1993

Clarkin JF, Widiger TA, Frances A, et al: Prototypic typology and the borderline personality disorder. J Abnorm Psychol 92:263–275, 1983

Cloninger CR: A systematic method for clinical description and classification of personality variants. Arch Gen Psychiatry 44:579–588, 1987

Cloninger CR, Svrakic DM, Pryzbeck TR: A psychobiological model of temperament and characters. Arch Gen Psychiatry 50:975–990, 1993

Coccaro EF: Psychopharmacologic studies in patients with personality disorders: review and perspective. Journal of Personality Disorders 7(suppl):181–192, 1993

Coccaro EF, Kavoussi RJ: Fluoxetine and impulsive aggressive behavior in personality-disordered subjects. Arch Gen Psychiatry 54:1081–1088, 1997

Coccaro EF, Siever L, Klar HM, et al: Serotonergic studies in patients with affective and personality disorders: correlates with suicidal and impulsive behaviors. Arch Gen Psychiatry 46:587–599, 1989

Coccaro EF, Harvey PD, Kupsaw-Lawrence E, et al: Development of neuropharmacologically based behavioral assessments of impulsive aggressive behavior. Journal of Neuropsychiatry 3:S44–S51, 1991

Costa PT, McRae RR: From catalog to Murray's needs and the five factor model. J Pers Soc Psychol 55:258–265, 1988

Cowdry RW, Gardner DL: Pharmacotherapy of borderline personality disorder: alprazolam, carbamazepine, trifluoperazine, and tranylcypromine. Arch Gen Psychiatry 45:111–119, 1988

Cowdry RW, Gardner DL, O'Leary KM: Mood variability: a study of four groups. Am J Psychiatry 148:1505–1511, 1991

de la Fuente JM, Lotstra F: A trial of carbamazepine in borderline personality disorder. Eur Neuropsychopharmacol 4:479–486, 1994

Deltito JA, Stam M: Psychopharmacological treatment of avoidant personality disorder. Compr Psychiatry 30:498–504, 1989

Department of Health, Education, and Welfare: Abnormal Involuntary Movements Scale. Washington, DC, U.S. Department of Health, Education, and Welfare

Depue RA, Slater JF, Wolfstetter-Kausch H, et al: A behavioral paradigm for identifying persons at risk for bipolar depressive disorder: a conceptual framework and five validation studies. J Abnorm Psychol 90:381–437, 1981

Derogatis LR, Lipman RS, Rickels K, et al: The Hopkins Symptom Checklist (HSCL): a self-report symptom inventory. Behav Sci 19:1–15, 1974

Dunn GE, Poalo AM, Ryan JJ, et al: Dissociative symptoms in a substance abuse population. Am J Psychiatry 150:1043–1047, 1993

Endicott J, Spitzer RL, Fleiss JL, et al: The Global Assessment Scale: a procedure for measuring overall severity of psychiatric disturbance. Arch Gen Psychiatry 33:766–771, 1976

Fahlen T: Personality traits in social phobia, II: changes during drug treatment. J Clin Psychiatry 56:569–573, 1995

Fleishhacker WW, Bergmann KJ, Perovich R, et al: The Hillside Akathisia Scale: a new rating instrument for neuroleptic induced akathisia. Psychopharmacol Bull 25:222–226, 1989

Folstein MF, Luria R: Reliability, validity, and clinical application of the Visual Analogue Mood Scale. Psychol Med 3:479–486, 1973

Gitlin MJ: Pharmacotherapy of personality disorders: conceptual framework and clinical strategies. J Clin Psychopharmacol 13:343–353, 1993

Gunderson JG, Phillips KA: A current view of the interface between borderline personality disorder and depression. Am J Psychiatry 148:967–975, 1991

Gunderson JG, Frank AF, Ronningstam EF, et al: Early discontinuance of borderline patients from psychotherapy. J Nerv Ment Dis 177:38–42, 1989

Gunderson JG, Zanarini M, Cassandra L: Borderline personality disorder: a review of the data on DSM-III-R descriptions. Journal of Personality Disorders 5:340–352, 1991

Gunderson JG, Links PS: Borderline personality disorder, in Treatments of Psychiatric Disorders, 2nd Edition. Edited by Gabbard GO. Washington, DC, American Psychiatric Press, 1995, pp 2291–2309

Guyatt G, Sackett D, Adachi J, et al: A clinician's guide for conducting randomized trials in individual patients. Can Med Assoc J 139:497–503, 1988

Harvey PD, Greenberg BR, Serper MR: The affective lability scales: development, reliability, and validity. J Clin Psychol 45:786–793, 1989

Hogan TP, Awad AG, Eastwood MR: A self-report scale predictive of drug compliance in schizophrenia: reliability and discriminative validity. Psychol Med 13:177–183, 1983

Hollifield M, Katon W, Skipper B, et al: Panic disorder and quality of life: variables predictive of functional impairment. Am J Psychiatry 154:766–772, 1997

Howard KI, Kopta SM, Krause M, et al: The dose-effect relationship in psychotherapy. Am Psychol 41:159–164, 1986

Iannaccone S, Ferini-Strambi L: Pharmacologic treatment of emotional lability. Clin Neuropharmacol 19:532–535, 1996

Joffe RT, Regan JJ: Personality and depression. J Psychiatr Res 22:279–286, 1988

Kavoussi RJ, Liu J, Coccaro EF: An open trial of sertraline in personality disordered patients with impulsive aggression. J Clin Psychiatry 55:137–141, 1994

Kay S, Opler L, Lindenmayer J: The positive and negative symptom syndrome scale (PANSS): rationale and standardization. Br J Psychiatry 155(suppl):59–65, 1989

Kelly T, Soloff PH, Cornelius J, et al: Can we study (treat) borderline patients? attrition from research and open treatment. Journal of Personality Disorders 6:417–433, 1992

Kernberg O: Borderline Conditions and Pathological Narcissism. New York, Jason Aronson, 1975

Koenigsberg HW: The role of medication in the treatment of borderline personality disorder, in Supportive Therapy for Borderline Patients. Edited by Rockland LH. New York, Guilford, 1992, pp 254–268

Kopta SM, Howard KI, Lowry JL, et al: Patterns of symptomatic recovery in psychotherapy. J Consult Clin Psychol 62:1009–1016, 1994

Lehman AF: The well-being of chronic mental patients. Arch Gen Psychiatry 40:369–373, 1983

Lehman AF, Ward NC, Linn LS: Chronic mental patients. Am J Psychiatry 139:1271–1276, 1982

Lehman AF, Possidente S, Hawker F: The quality of life of chronic patients in a state hospital and in community residences. Hosp Comm Psychiatry 37:901–907, 1986

Lenzenweger MF, Clarkin JF: The personality disorders: history, classification, and research issues, in Major Theories of Personality Disorder. Edited by Clarkin JF, Lenzenweger MF. New York, Guilford, 1996, pp 1–35

Liebowitz MR, Schneier F, Campeas R, et al: Phenelzine vs. atenolol in social phobia: a placebo-controlled comparison. Arch Gen Psychiatry 49:290–300, 1992

Lienemann J, Walker F: Naltrexone for treatment of self-injury. Am J Psychiatry 146:1639–1640, 1989

Linehan M, Armstrong H, Suarez A, et al: Cognitive-behavioral treatment of chronically parasuicidal borderline patients. Arch Gen Psychiatry 48:1060–1064, 1991

Links PS: Psychiatric rehabilitation model for borderline personality disorder. Can J Psychiatry 38:S35–S38, 1993

Links PS: Comprehending comorbidity: a symptom disorder plus a personality disorder, in Clinical Assessment and Management of Severe Personality Disorders. Edited by Links PS. Washington, DC, American Psychiatric Press, 1996, pp 93–108

Links PS, Steiner M: Psychopharmacologic management of patients with borderline personality disorder. Can J Psychiatry 33:355–359, 1988

Links PS, Steiner M, Offord DR, et al: Characteristics of borderline personality disorder: a Canadian sample. Can J Psychiatry 33:336–340, 1988

Links PS, Boiago I, Huxley G, et al: Sexual abuse and biparental failure as etiologic models in borderline personality disorder, in Family Environment and Borderline Personality Disorder. Edited by Links PS. Washington, DC, American Psychiatric Press, 1990a, pp 105–120

Links PS, Steiner M, Boiago I, et al: Lithium therapy for borderline patients: preliminary findings. Journal of Personality Disorders 4:173–181, 1990b

Links PS, Heslegrave RJ, Mitton JE, et al: Borderline personality disorder and substance abuse: consequences of comorbidity. Can J Psychiatry 40:9–14, 1995

Links PS, Boiago I, Allnutt S: Understanding and recognizing personality disorders, in Clinical Assessment and Management of Severe Personality Disorders. Edited by Links PS. Washington, DC, American Psychiatric Press, 1996, pp 1–19

Little K, Penman E: Measuring subacute mood changes using the profile of mood states and visual analogue scales. Psychopathology 22:42–49, 1989

Livesley WJ, Jang KL, Jackson DN, et al: Genetic and environmental contributions to dimensions of personality disorder. Am J Psychiatry 150:1826–1831, 1993

Markowitz PJ, Calabrese JR, Schulz SC, et al: Fluoxetine in the treatment of borderline and schizotypal personality disorders. Am J Psychiatry 148:1064–1067, 1991

McGee MD: Cessation of self-mutilation in a patient with borderline personality disorder treated with naltrexone. J Clin Psychiatry 58:32–33, 1997

McGlashan TH: The prediction of outcome in borderline personality disorder: part V of the Chestnut Lodge follow-up study, in The Borderline: Current Empirical Research. Edited by McGlashan TH. Washington, DC, American Psychiatric Press, 1985, pp 61–98

Montgomery AS, Montgomery D: Pharmacological prevention of suicidal behavior. J Affective Disord 4:291–298, 1982

Nakao K, Gunderson JG, Phillips KA, et al: Functional impairment in personality disorders. Journal of Personality Disorders 6:24–33, 1992

Norton GR, Ross CA, Novotny MF: Factors that predict scores on the Dissociative Experiences Scale. J Clin Psychol 46:273–277, 1990

Nurnberg G, Raskin M, Levine PE, et al: The comorbidity of borderline personality disorder with other DSM-III-R Axis II personality disorders. Am J Psychiatry 148:1311–1317, 1991

O'Malley SS, Jaffe AJ, Chang G, et al: Naltrexone and coping skills therapy for alcohol dependence. Arch Gen Psychiatry 49:881–887, 1992

Paris J: Social Factors in Personality Disorders: A Biopsychosocial Approach to Etiology and Treatment. Cambridge, UK, Cambridge University Press, 1996

Paris J, Brown R, Nowlis D: Long-term follow-up of borderline patients in a general hospital. Compr Psychiatry 28:530–535, 1987

Perry JC: Problems and considerations in the valid assessments of personality disorders. Am J Psychiatry 149:1645–1653, 1992

Pfohl B, Coryell W, Zimmerman M, et al: DSM-III personality disorders: diagnostic overlap and internal consistency of individual DSM-III criteria. Compr Psychiatry 27:21–34, 1986

Plomin R: The role of inheritance in behavior. Science 248:183–188, 1990

Reich J, Noyes R Jr, Yates W: Alprazolam treatment of avoidant personality traits in social phobic patients. J Clin Psychiatry 50:91–95, 1989

Roth AS, Ostroff RB, Hoffman RE: Naltrexone as a treatment for repetitive self-injurious behavior: an open-label trial. J Clin Psychiatry 57:233–237, 1996

Rutter M: Temperament, personality, and personality development. Br J Psychiatry 150:443–448, 1987

Schou M: Forty years of lithium treatment. Arch Gen Psychiatry 54:9–13, 1997

Sherbourne CD, Wells KB, Meredith LS, et al: Comorbid anxiety disorder and the functioning and well-being of chronically ill patients of general medical providers. Arch Gen Psychiatry 53:889–895, 1996

Siever LS, Davis KL: A psychobiologic perspective on the personality disorders. Am J Psychiatry 148:1647–1658, 1991

Silk KR: Rational pharmacotherapy for patients with personality disorders, in Clinical Assessment and Management of Severe Personality Disorders. Edited by Links PS. Washington, DC, American Psychiatric Press, 1996, pp 109–142

Soloff PH: What's new in personality disorders? an update on pharmacologic treatment. Journal of Personality Disorders 4:233–243, 1990

Soloff PH: Pharmacological therapies in borderline personality disorder, in Borderline Personality Disorder: Etiology and Treatment. Edited by Paris J. Washington, DC, American Psychiatric Press, 1993, pp 319–348

Soloff PH: Symptom-oriented psychopharmacology for personality disorders. Journal of Practical Psychiatry and Behavioral Health (in press)

Soloff PH, George A, Nathan RS, et al: Progress in the pharmacotherapy of borderline disorders: a double-blind study of amitriptyline, haloperidol, and placebo. Arch Gen Psychiatry 43:691–697, 1986

Soloff PH, Cornelius J, George A, et al: Efficacy of phenelzine and haloperidol in borderline personality disorder. Arch Gen Psychiatry 50:377–385, 1993

Stein DJ, Simeon D, Frenkel M, et al: An open trial of valproate in borderline personality disorder. J Clin Psychiatry 56:506–510, 1995

Steinberg M, Rounsaville B, Cicchetti D: Detection of dissociative disorders in psychiatric patients by a screening instrument and a structured diagnostic interview. Am J Psychiatry 148:1050–1054, 1991

Stone MH: The Fate of Borderline Patients. New York, Guilford, 1990

van Ameringen M, Mancini C, Streiner DL: Fluoxetine efficacy in social phobia. J Clin Psychiatry 54:27–32, 1993

van Ameringen M, Mancini C, Streiner D: Sertraline in social phobia. J Affective Disord 31:141–145, 1994

van der Kolk BA: Traumatic Stress: The Effects of Overwhelming Experience on Mind, Body, and Society. New York, Guilford, 1996

van Reekum R, Links PS: N of 1 study: methylphenidate in a patient with borderline personality disorder and attention deficit hyperactivity disorder (letter). Can J Psychiatry 39:186–187, 1994

van Reekum R, Links PS, Boiago I: Constitutional factors in borderline personality disorder: genetics, brain dysfunction, and biological markers, in Borderline Personality Disorder: Etiology and Treatment. Edited by Paris J. Washington, DC, American Psychiatric Press, 1993, pp 13–38

van Reekum R, Links PS, Fedorov C: Impulsivity in borderline personality disorder, in Biological and Neurobehavioral Studies of Borderline Personality Disorder. Edited by Silk KR. Washington, DC, American Psychiatric Press, 1994, pp 1–22

Versiani M, Nardi AE, Mundim FD, et al: Pharmacotherapy of social phobia: a controlled study with moclobemide and phenelzine. Br J Psychiatry 161:353–360, 1992

Volpicelli JR, Alterman AI, Hayashida M, et al: Naltrexone in the treatment of alcohol dependence. Arch Gen Psychiatry 49:876–880, 1992

Waldinger R, Gunderson JG: Completed psychotherapies with borderline patients. Am J Psychother 38:190–202, 1984

Waller DA, Kiser RS, Hardy BW, et al: Eating behavior and plasma beta-endorphin in bulimia. Am J Clin Nutr 44:20–23, 1986

Westen D: Divergences between clinical and research methods for assessing personality disorders: implications for research and evolution of Axis II. Am J Psychiatry 154:895–903, 1997

Wilcox JA: Divalproex sodium as a treatment for borderline personality disorder. Ann Clin Psychiatry 7:33–37, 1995

Willemsen-Swinkels SHN, Buitelaar KJ, Nijhof GJ, et al: Failure of naltrexone hydrochloride to reduce self-injurious and autistic behavior in mentally retarded adults. Arch Gen Psychiatry 52:766–773, 1995

Winchel RM, Stanley M: Self-injurious behavior: a review of the behavior and biology of self-mutilation. Am J Psychiatry 148:306–317, 1991

Chapter 5

Significance of Biological Research for a Biopsychosocial Model of the Personality Disorders

Joel Paris, M.D.

Etiological Models and Personality Disorders

Personality disorders are complex forms of psychopathology that cannot be accounted for using simple causal explanations. Understanding the pathways from normal to abnormal personality requires the use of multidimensional models that take into account biological, psychological, and social factors.

The biopsychosocial model (Engel 1980) assumes that constitution, experience, and the social environment are all crucial in the etiology of mental disorders. However, their contributions need not be equal. There are, in fact, good reasons to consider biological factors as having a privileged role in psychopathology. Genetic predispositions determine which kinds of disorder individuals may develop, whereas psychosocial factors function as precipitants of pathology (Cloninger et al. 1990). This approach, which corresponds to the *diathesis-stress model* of mental disorders (Monroe and Simons 1991), suggests that genes shape predispositions and environmental stressors determine whether underlying vulnerabilities develop into overt disorders.

The diathesis-stress model can also be seen as following logically from the principles of quantitative genetics (Falconer 1989). Thus, predispositions for most forms of disease involve many gene loci. Interactions between these loci yield a normal distribution of traits. Disease develops only when the combined weight of predispositions and stressors exceeds a given threshold.

These principles apply to most forms of psychiatric illness (Paris, in press). In common mental disorders such as schizophrenia, depression, or substance use, the number of individuals developing disorders is far exceeded by those who carry predispositions, and environmental precipitants are usually thought to be required to produce overt pathology. The nature of these precipitants ranges from the intrauterine brain insults implicated in schizophrenia (Weinberger 1987) to the interpersonal losses that can be precipitants of depression (Paykel and Cooper 1992) and to the social pressures that encourage substance use (Helzer and Canino 1992).

The diathesis-stress model is particularly applicable to the personality disorders. The diatheses for these conditions are trait profiles. Traits determine what kinds of disorders will probably develop, and when these traits are unusually intense, they may be risk factors for pathology (Siever and Davis 1991). The stressors that can elicit personality disorders range widely from psychological adversities to social disintegration (Paris 1996).

Temperament and Traits

The biological predispositions shaping normal and abnormal personality consist of variations in temperament (Rutter 1987b). *Temperament* can be defined in terms of behavioral propensities present at birth. Individuals vary quite widely in inborn characteristics, but these differences, by themselves, need not lead to dysfunction.

In a well-known study (Chess and Thomas 1984), normal children whose temperaments were measured at birth were followed into young adulthood. On follow-up, there were surprisingly few continuities between infant temperament and adult personality. Even the most consistent correlation, between a "difficult" temperament and problems in adulthood, was not strong enough to allow clinical prediction of psychopathology (Chess and Thomas 1990).

In recent years, research has shifted from normal populations to the long-term follow-up studies of infants with abnormal temperaments. The most important of these studies, by Maziade et al. (1990) and Kagan (1994), examined cohorts who have now reached adolescence. Maziade and colleagues studied infants with high levels of irritability, a temperamental characteristic that could be a precursor of a number of personality disorders, particularly in the dramatic cluster. Kagan's group studied infants with extreme social anxiety ("behavioral inhibition") that could be precursors for personality disorders in the anxious cluster.

In adults, temperament is measured indirectly through the assessment of *traits*, the enduring patterns of behavior that characterize individual differences in personality. Genetic factors account for nearly half of the variance in explaining individual differences in traits (Plomin et al. 1997).

Behavioral genetic findings also show that more than half of the variance in personality derives from environmental factors. The nature of the environmental influence on personality may come as something of a surprise (Reiss et al. 1992). Instead of deriving largely from growing up in a particular family (a " 'shared' component"), the environmental component depends on a wide range of experiences unique to the individual (an " 'unshared' component"). Although parents do not always treat siblings equally, differential rearing is often a function of the child's temperament (Chess and Thomas 1984). In any case, the greater importance of unshared environment presents a clear challenge to traditional theories claiming that parental practices are the primary factors shaping personality development.

The sources or sites of the unshared environmental influence on personality could derive from many roots and routes: differential treatment of siblings, congruence or incongruence of traits between parents and children, birth order effects (Sulloway 1996), and trait differences leading to different perceptions of the same environment (Kendler and Eaves 1986), as well as from the impact of life experiences outside of the family.

The magnitude of the effects associated with unique environmental factors indicates that although temperamental factors "bend the twig," they do not, by themselves, determine the shape of the entire tree (i.e., decide individual differences in trait profiles). Nonetheless, it seems unlikely that environmental factors could ever be strong enough to completely reverse trait dispositions. Thus, as suggested by Kagan (1994), externalizing symptoms are most likely to develop in children who are temperamentally impulsive, while internalizing symptoms are much more commonly seen in children who are temperamentally anxious. In each of these scenarios, environmental factors, rather than acting as primary causal factors, amplify temperamental dispositions.

Personality Traits and Personality Disorders

Personality disorders are pathological *amplifications* of normal traits (Paris 1996). This theoretical principle is supported by evidence from both clinical and community populations (Livesley et al. 1992), pointing to strong continuities between traits and disorders. This continuity model is also consistent with the threshold model of disease discussed earlier.

In view of these continuities, some theorists (Costa and Widiger 1994) have suggested replacing the current Axis II system of categories with a dimensional system. However, dimensions, such as those described in the five-factor model, or in the Cloninger system (Cloninger 1987), are not sufficiently meaningful to practitioners, who prefer to describe clinical prototypes (Westen 1997).

An alternative approach involves the description of personality pathology using dimensions derived from the study of patients with personality disorders. For example, in a system developed at Mount Sinai School of Medicine in New York City (Siever and Davis 1991), four dimensions (impulsive, affective, anxious, and cognitive) are proposed to define the traits that underlie disorders. Similarly, a system developed at the University of British Columbia in Vancouver (Livesley et al. 1992) uses 18 dimensions describing various forms of personality pathology that can then be grouped into four higher-order factors (lability, antagonism, interpersonal unresponsiveness, and compulsivity). At present, researchers might best be advised to use both systems: a categorical approach is useful in describing clinically meaningful entities and a dimensional approach is useful in making a clearer separation between symptomatic presentations.

One might expect that if traits are heritable, then the disorders that derive from them should also demonstrate strong genetic influence. However, heritability is not a characteristic of individuals but rather of populations. At the extreme ends of a continuum, traits could show either more or less genetic influence (Nigg and Goldsmith 1994). Little systematic research has been conducted in this area, with what evidence there is suggesting that personality disorders are less heritable than normal traits (McGuffin and Thapar 1992; Nigg and Goldsmith 1994). These findings are consistent with the hypothesis that trait amplification is driven by psychosocial environmental factors.

Applying a stress-diathesis model, trait profiles would be the diatheses that determine what type of personality disorder any individual can develop (Paris 1996). These mechanisms can be clarified by returning to the contrast between impulsive and anxious traits. Only those with trait impulsivity would be expected to develop impulsive personality disorders on Axis II, such as antisocial or borderline personality disorder (BPD). In contrast, individuals with anxious temperaments would not be expected to develop these disorders, which are characterized by low thresholds for risk-taking behaviors (i.e., impulsivity). Similarly, only those with trait anxiety would be expected to develop anxious personality disorders on Axis II, such as avoidant or obsessive-compulsive personality disorders. In contrast, individuals with impulsive temperaments would not be expected to develop these anxious disorders, which are characterized by high thresholds for risk-taking behaviors.

Social Factors in the Personality Disorders

Personality traits are alternative strategies for adaptation to environmental demands (Beck and Freeman 1990). Therefore, there is room in the world for a multitude of personality types, each of which can be adaptive or maladaptive under different conditions.

Applying Eysenck's (1991) schema, extroverts are better at building social networks but run the danger of excessive dependence on validation from other people. Introverts are better at focusing on tasks and may function better in low-stimulation environments but run the danger of becoming isolated. Individuals with high levels of neuroticism dissipate energy in unnecessary worry, whereas those with low levels of neuroticism may be insufficiently vigilant under conditions of environmental threat.

Similar considerations apply to the three additional dimensions introduced in the five-factor model (Costa and Widiger 1994). Individuals who are highly open to experience have the advantage of imaginativeness but the disadvantage of overly permeable personal boundaries. Individuals who are highly agreeable may please others but fail to please themselves. Individuals who are highly conscientious may be productive but can easily become grounded or stuck by their high standards. In Cloninger's (1987) schema, too much novelty seeking creates instability, whereas too little is associated with rigidity; too much harm avoidance leads to anxiety, whereas too little leads to impulsivity; too much reward dependence makes people excessively agreeable, whereas too little makes them disagreeable.

The degree of adaptiveness of any trait is relative to social context. When cultures change, one might expect age cohort effects to influence the prevalence of different traits in the changed culture. Depending on the social structure, there should also be cross-cultural differences in personality trait profiles. Research confirms the expectation of cross-cultural differences. Although the same personality structures can be found in different countries (McCrae and Costa 1997), there are measurable differences on personality dimensions among societies (Eysenck 1991). Although such differences could be partly attributable to ethnic differences in temperament, they are most likely cultural.

Epidemiological studies of the prevalence of personality disorders have also demonstrated cohort effects and cross-cultural differences, particularly for antisocial personality. This form of pathology has increased dramatically in North America over the last several decades (Robins and Regier 1991). Although the precise reasons for this cohort change are not known, the risk factors for antisocial behavior include major family dysfunction (Robins 1966) and social disintegration (Paris 1996).

Findings concerning cross-cultural differences in the prevalence of antisocial personality are particularly provocative. This diagnosis remains quite rare in Taiwan (Hwu et al. 1989), as well as in Japan (Sato and Takeichi 1993). These two societies, which are highly cohesive and have family and social structures that Westerners consider authoritarian, encourage the suppression of emotional displays and impulsive actions. Yet even in East Asia, Confucian traits are not universal, as shown by the high rates of both alcoholism and antisocial personality disorder in the very different society of South Korea (Lee et al. 1987).

Indirect evidence suggests that, similar to antisocial personality disorder, BPD may be relatively uncommon in traditional societies. In particular, behaviors associated with impulsivity and affective instability, such as self-mutilation and suicide attempts, are much more frequent in societies undergoing modernization, particularly when social change is unusually rapid (Paris 1994).

Linehan's (1993) biosocial model of BPD hypothesizes interactions between heritable traits and social structures that lead to borderline pathology. In her view, children likely to develop BPD later in life have a constitutionally determined emotional instability, characterized by a stronger emotional reaction to negative events and a longer time required to return to baseline after the event has passed. This concept of the temperamental vulnerability to borderline pathology, which resembles those of neuroticism and affective lability, differs from Siever and Davis's (1991) theoretical formulation, which sees impulsivity not as a separate dimension but as a secondary response. Linehan also hypothesizes that affectively unstable children require more buffering to help them modulate and control their dysphoric emotions. In this view, BPD develops out of interactions between temperamental factors and a lack of environmental responsiveness, what

Linehan (1993) calls an "invalidating environment." Linehan suggests that the modern world, which demands greater individual autonomy and allows less dependence on or attachment to others, interferes with the ability of children with stronger emotional needs to obtain sufficient care from their families.

Implications for Biological Research on Personality Disorders

Studies of the biological factors in personality disorders need to be conducted at an optimal level of analysis. In theory, personality should be closely linked to temperament. Moreover, both genetic and biological markers are more closely linked to traits than to disorders (Nigg and Goldsmith 1994). Thus, if we had purely temperamental measures, we would expect them to be strongly linked to biological markers and to specific gene loci. However, given the strong environmental factors influencing the development of personality, biological studies of normal traits can provide only approximate associations rather than specific correlates.

Furthermore, it appears unlikely that temperamental variations can be reduced to the activity levels of a limited number of neurotransmitters. The heritable component of personality, like most characteristics showing wide differences between individuals, is influenced by complex interactions between many genes. Each of these pathways may be quite complex, with single transmitters being affected by more than one gene and with single genes affecting more than one transmitter system. What we already know is that each neurotransmitter acts on several different receptor types, each of which has a different effect on behavior (Coccaro and Murphy 1990).

Moreover, the effects of individual neurotransmitters can be entirely different, even contradictory, at different sites of the brain. Transmitter systems have to be understood in the context of neuroanatomy and neurophysiology. Recently, with the development of brain imaging (Goyer et al. 1994) and the revival of neuropsychological research (O'Leary and Cowdry 1994), interest has been renewed in the localization of neural phenomena related to the personality disorders. For example, it may be just as important to determine that executive functions, located in the frontal lobe, are compromised in patients with impulsive personality disorders as it is to document changes in serotonergic activity.

It is therefore unlikely that researchers will ever find one-to-one correspondence between personality traits and biological markers. We are more likely to succeed in demonstrating that biological profiles have a consistent statistical relationship to personality. Similarly, it seems unlikely that research will identify simple correspondences between personality traits and genetic markers. It is possible that some genetic loci, such as that purported to be associated with novelty seeking (Benjamin et al. 1996), might account for some degree of temperamental variance. However, to identify individuals with temperamental characteristics that place them at risk for personality disorders, we may need to read the entire genome.

Theoretical and research programs to find specific biological correlates for personality traits or disorders are limited by our present level of knowledge about the brain. We need to know more about brain neurochemistry, and we then need to place that knowledge in the context of neuroanatomy and neurochemistry. These advances in basic research will lead us to define both traits and disorders in a new way, a way firmly based on biological variations. However, to do so at our present state of knowledge is not possible and can only be considered as heuristic.

Gene-Environment Interactions in Personality Disorders

Behavioral genetic research, somewhat paradoxically, provides important insight into the role of the environment. Kendler and Eaves (1986) have described two basic mechanisms of gene-environment interaction. In the first, genetic variability determines *susceptibility* to the environment. As documented later, the same environmental circumstances that may bring on pathology in some individuals have only minimal effects in others. In the second mechanism, genetic factors influence *exposure* to environmental risk factors. For example, temperamental characteristics, such as impulsivity, produce behaviors that make negative reactions from peers and caretakers much more likely (Rutter and Quinton 1984) or increase the likelihood that individuals will expose themselves to dangerous situations (Lyons et al. 1993).

We can apply these principles to understanding the role of environmental factors in personality disorders. Let us consider, for example, associations between psychological risks (trauma, loss, or emotional neglect) and impulsive personality disorders (Paris 1994, 1996). These findings have become well known among clinicians; less well known are the implications of studies that assess the impact of these same risk factors in community populations. For example, child abuse has been claimed to be a major factor in the etiology of BPD (Herman and van der Kolk 1987) and is clearly a risk factor for later psychiatric or psychological problems (Fergusson et al. 1996). Yet most adults who have experienced childhood sexual abuse (Browne and Finkelhor 1986) or childhood physical abuse (Malinovsky-Rummell and Hansen 1993) fail to show *any* psychological symptoms; only about 20% of those exposed to trauma develop demonstrable psychopathology. Interestingly, similar findings apply to traumatic events during adult life; only a vulnerable 25% of those exposed to the traumatic event develop symptoms (Yehuda and McFarlane 1995), while posttraumatic stress disorder itself has a strong heritable component (True et al. 1993).

These findings of not everyone who is exposed to trauma developing serious symptoms, as they apply to children, are in accord with the well-established principle of *resilience*. The majority of children show a surprising ability to bounce back from a wide variety of negative experiences (Rutter 1987a). Although a broad range of factors from both genetic and environmental sources shape resilience (Werner and Smith 1992), the most important factors appear to be intelligence and positive personality characteristics, both of which are influenced by genetics. These findings help to explain why adverse environmental factors have different effects on children with different temperaments. Similar conclusions apply to the impact of negative life events in adults (Kendler and Eaves 1986). In general, single adversities do not produce psychopathology, while multiple adversities have a cumulative effect that overwhelms natural resilience (Rutter 1987a).

The following general conclusions follow from these principles:

1. Biological factors in the personality disorders shape a temperamental matrix that increases the likelihood of pathological interactions with significant others in the environment.
2. Certain specific combinations of traits may be particularly likely to lead to these cascade effects of pathological temperament-environmental interactions.
3. Nonetheless, positive traits can buffer negative traits, and it is this buffering effect on the temperament-environmental interaction that may explain why most children are resilient to adversity.
4. Even in the presence of temperamental risk, protective factors associated with a positive environment can make the development of personality disorders much less likely.
5. Conversely, individuals without a significant temperamental risk can still develop personality disorders if exposed to continuous and cumulative "environmental" adversities.

Clinical Implications

Biological research on the personality disorders could lead to three possible directions for future clinical practice. The first concerns the possibility of developing new forms of pharmacological treatment for patients with personality disorders. The second involves the possibility of gene therapy. The third involves new forms of psychotherapy based on a better understanding of temperament.

At present, drug treatment in patients with personality disorders is ubiquitous yet not particularly effective. Controlled studies may show more success than actual clinical practice.

Drug trials in patients with BPD have had rather discouraging results (Soloff 1993), with positive findings being either clinically marginal or unsustained over time. Moreover, attempts to carry out "pharmacological dissection" of personality pathology into component traits that could be the target of biological intervention have not yet proved fruitful (Soloff 1993), though attempts are being made to develop algorithms and other pharmacological treatment strategies that may eventually prove useful (Soloff, in press) (see Chapter 4 of this text). On the whole, theories of the neurochemical basis of personality disorders are not fully in accord with pharmacological findings. Each neurochemical system is highly complex, and each pathway interacts with many others. Thus, although it has been suggested that patients with impulsive personality disorders have a sluggish serotonergic system (Coccaro et al. 1989 [also see Chapter 1 of this text]), and some clinical trials suggest that some patients improve with specific serotonin reuptake inhibitors (Markowitz 1995), these effects are much less consistent and far less dramatic than those seen in patients with melancholic depression (Gunderson and Phillips 1991; Soloff 1993). Effective drugs for personality disorders may belong not to the future rather than the present. Research is needed to develop agents with specific effects on impulsivity as well as on affective instability.

Gene therapy for mental disorders may be pure science fiction at present, but it is conceivable that such intervention could become a normative part of practice in the coming century. However, since traits are influenced by multiple genes, it is difficult to imagine that personality disorders could be treated in the same way as purely genetic diseases. The only practical scenario would be to target single genes that account for a significant percentage of the variance in a trait and that produce a cascade effect through their interactions with other genetic and environmental factors.

The third possibility concerns developing new forms of psychotherapy, which has immediate practical application. Trait theory provides a scientific basis for the traditional nostrum that different folks need different strokes.

Cognitive-behavioral therapists, who are known for a willingness to experiment, have been particularly energetic in applying these principles. Beck and Freeman (1990) have proposed a model for therapy of personality disorders individualized according to the traits underlying each form of disorder. Unfortunately, these ideas have not yet generated research demonstrating that the methods derived from theory are indeed effective.

Linehan's (1993) treatment program for BPD is also based on a diathesis-stress model that takes into account the temperamental abnormalities underlying this form of pathology. The treatment is based on the idea that cognitive and behavioral interventions can reshape traits into more adaptive directions. Thus, recognizing the importance of biology in personality disorders need not lead clinicians to focus exclusively on psychopharmacological interventions.

Paris (1998) has offered a similar general model of the personality disorders that combines psychodynamic and behavioral theories and methods. By taking trait profiles into account, therapy can help patients to reverse trait amplification and thus make better use of underlying traits. This approach can be thought of as a clinical application of the theory of gene-environment interactions in personality development.

The following case examples (for details, see Paris 1998) demonstrate some of these theoretical mechanisms.

Case 1: Borderline Personality Disorder

Suzanne was a 22-year-old teacher who presented with suicidal ideas, auditory hallucinations, and chronic mood swings. She also suffered from dissociative states in which she would break into uncontrollable crying spells for hours at a time and then begin to hear voices.

Suzanne was described by her mother as an energetic child who had always been a "handful" and who needed to be watched to prevent her from getting into trouble. These temperamental characteristics stood in contrast to those of her younger sister, who had always been placid and easy to manage. From adolescence, Suzanne developed unstable and problematic relationships, while her sister held a steady course in life by becoming a professional and marrying her first boyfriend.

Both sisters had suffered from being raised by parents who were chronically estranged and unable to attend to their children's or each other's emotional needs. However, Suzanne was more affected by the situation, especially when her mother left the family to live with a lover. Her mother took the children back the following year only because the father moved to Europe for business reasons. Suzanne came to depend on the one sure method she had learned for obtaining the attention she lacked at home. Boys saw her as lively and sexy, and she found that she got a "kick" out of seducing as many of them as possible.

In treatment, Suzanne was initially given two pharmacological agents: neuroleptics to help her to stop hearing voices and a serotonin reuptake inhibitor to control her moods. Antidepressants had little impact on her symptoms, but Suzanne kept a low-dose neuroleptic on hand, since it was generally effective in aborting her dissociative spells.

Psychotherapy helped Suzanne to avoid suppressing inner feelings, which would build to the point of eruption and lead to either impulsive actions or spells. Suzanne therefore learned to pay attention to her emotions on a daily basis. Practicing these skills helped her to avoid having "affective storms."

Suzanne's impulsivity and affective lability, however much they created problems, had a potentially positive side. She was an active and lively woman with good sense of humor. People often took to Suzanne, so that she never lacked for friends. Although she learned to control her self-destructive impulses, she remained action oriented and highly emotional. These traits had proved to be adaptive in her work as a teacher, and one of the first goals of treatment was to get her back to work as soon as possible.

Case 2: Avoidant Personality Disorder

Cora was a 40-year-old family doctor who presented for treatment because of her inability to live with another person in an intimate relationship. Although she was afraid of rejection, she also felt intolerably confined by intimacy.

Cora had been an unusually shy child who suffered from high levels of stranger anxiety and who had always had difficulty relating to her peer group. Throughout her life, Cora felt anxious in groups and always sought safety in one-to-one contact with intimates whom she had known for years.

Cora was brought up in a large family in which the parents

were overwhelmed by their children's needs. For a time, Cora was sent to live with her aunt and uncle in a nearby town. However, since she was bright, she could compensate for the lack of affection in her family by doing well academically, and she became the favorite of the nuns teaching at her school.

Cora was a cautious woman with a strong need to control her environment. Her personality was adaptive for working as a physician, a task that required her to investigate complex clinical problems. She had been working for many years at the same clinic, and her co-workers had become "like family" to her. In this milieu, she could obtain validation without sacrificing space. Cora began to have love affairs in her 30s, but they were largely unsatisfactory, and she felt she was missing out on the satisfactions other people found in life.

Cora had previously been treated with serotonin reuptake inhibitors but without visible effects. The work in psychotherapy aimed to help her find practical ways to overcome her trait anxiety. Through gradual exposure, she was able to find a relationship that offered a reasonable compromise between her needs for closeness and space. Eventually, she developed a long-term attachment to a single man, with the understanding that they had no need to live together. At the same time, her commitment to her work continued to provide her with meaningful satisfaction.

Discussion

Each of these clinical vignettes demonstrates the biopsychosocial determinants of personality disorders. In both cases, temperamental factors strongly influenced the nature of stable trait profiles and the type of personality disorder that eventually developed. Under stress, Suzanne's impulsive traits became amplified to the point that she developed seriously dysfunctional symptoms, most particularly impulsive actions, mood instability, and dissociation. Similarly, Cora's anxious traits became amplified to the point that she became paralyzed by the fear of rejection and was unable to establish intimate attachments in adult life.

Each of these cases also demonstrates how the treatment of personality disorders needs to be broadly multidimensional. Suzanne required intermittent use of medication, and although Cora did not respond to psychopharmacology, it remains possible that some patients with avoidant personality may benefit from selective serotonin reuptake inhibitors (Kramer 1993) or monoamine oxidase inhibitors (Liebowitz et al. 1992; Schneier et al. 1991). In each of these cases, eclectic psychotherapy tried to target maladaptive traits with the aim of reversing their amplification and also employed psychoeducational methods to help these patients to make better use of the positive aspects of their existing traits.

Conclusions

Biological research in the area of personality disorders has reached an exciting frontier. However, we need to remain humble and take a long view. Even in "the decade of the brain," the neurosciences are in a very primitive stage of development. As the basic sciences move forward, clinical science will be in a better position to advance.

We have come a long way from the days when personality traits and personality disorders were seen as almost exclusively the result of childhood experiences. This having been said, psychiatrists should be careful about jumping to the opposite conclusion that biology is the predominant factor in personality. If disorders are multidimensional, we need to carry out multidimensional research. Instead of studying biology and experience separately, we should try to develop methodologies to examine the interactions between biology and environment in the course of personality development.

References

Beck AT, Freeman A: Cognitive Therapy of Personality Disorders, New York, Guilford, 1990

Benjamin J, Patterson C, Greenberg BD, et al: Population and familial association between the D_4 receptor gene and measures of novelty seeking. Nat Genet 12:81–84, 1996

Browne A, Finkelhor D: Impact of child sexual abuse: a review of the literature. Psychol Bull 99:66–77, 1986

Chess S, Thomas A: Origins and Evolution of Behavior Disorders. New York, Brunner/Mazel, 1984

Chess S, Thomas A: The New York Longitudinal Study: the young adult periods. Can J Psychiatry 35:557–561, 1990

Cloninger CR: A systematic method for clinical description and classification of personality variants. Arch Gen Psychiatry 44:579–588, 1987

Cloninger CR, Martin RL, Guze SB, et al: The empirical structure of psychiatric comorbidity and its theoretical significance, in Comorbidity of Anxiety and Depression. Edited by Maser JD, Cloninger CR. Washington, DC, American Psychiatric Press, 1990, pp 439–462

Coccaro EF, Murphy DS (eds): Serotonin in Major Psychiatric Disorders. Washington, DC, American Psychiatric Press, 1990

Coccaro EF, Siever LJ, Klar HM, et al: Serotonergic studies in patients with affective and personality disorders. Arch Gen Psychiatry 46:587–599, 1989

Costa PT, Widiger TA (eds): Personality Disorders and the Five-Factor Model of Personality. Washington, DC, American Psychological Association, 1994

Engel GL: The clinical application of the biopsychosocial model. Am J Psychiatry 137:535–544, 1980

Eysenck HJ: Genetic and environmental contributions to individual differences: the three major dimensions of personality. J Pers 58:245–261, 1991

Falconer DS: Introduction to Quantitative Genetics. Essex, Longman, 1989

Fergusson DM, Lynskey MT, Horwood J: Childhood sexual abuse and psychiatric disorder in young adulthood, II: psychiatric outcomes of childhood sexual abuse. J Am Acad Child Adolesc Psychiatry 34:1365–1374, 1996

Goyer PF, Konicki PE, Schulz SC: Brain imaging in personality disorders, in Biological and Neurobehavioral Studies of Borderline Personality Disorder. Edited by Silk KR. Washington, DC, American Psychiatric Press, 1994, pp 109–127

Gunderson JG, Phillips KA: A current view of the interface between borderline personality disorder and depression. Am J Psychiatry 148:967–975, 1991

Helzer JE, Canino GJ (eds): Alcoholism in North America, Europe, and Asia. New York, Oxford University Press, 1992

Herman JL, van der Kolk BA: Traumatic antecedents of borderline personality disorder, in Psychological Trauma. Edited by van der Kolk BA. Washington, DC, American Psychiatric Press, 1987, pp 111–126

Hwu HG, Yeh EK, Change LY: Prevalence of psychiatric disorders in Taiwan defined by the Chinese Diagnostic Interview Schedule. Acta Psychiatr Scand 79:136–147, 1989

Kagan J: Galen's Prophecy. New York, Basic Books, 1994

Kendler KS, Eaves LJ: Models for the joint effect of genotype and environment on liability to psychiatric illness. Am J Psychiatry 143:279–289, 1986

Kramer P: Listening to Prozac. New York, Viking, 1993

Lee KC, Kovac YS, Rhee H: The national epidemiological study of mental disorders in Korea. J Korean Med Sci 2:19–34, 1987

Liebowitz MR, Schneier F, Campbell R, et al: Phenelzine vs. atenolol in social phobia: a placebo-controlled comparison. Arch Gen Psychiatry 49:290–300, 1992

Linehan MM: Cognitive Behavioral Treatment of Borderline Personality Disorder. New York, Guilford, 1993

Livesley WJ, Jackson DN, Schroeder ML: Factorial structure of traits delineating personality disorders in clinical and general population samples. J Abnorm Psychol 101:432–440, 1992

Lyons MJ, Goldberg J, Eisen SA, et al: Do genes influence exposure to trauma? a twin study of combat. Am J Med Genet 48:22–27, 1993

Malinovsky-Rummell R, Hansen DJ: Long-term consequences of physical abuse. Psychol Bull 114:68–79, 1993

Markowitz PJ: Pharmacotherapy of impulsivity, aggression, and related disorders, in Impulsivity and Aggression. Edited by Hollander E, Stein DJ. New York, Wiley, 1995, pp 263–286

Maziade M, Caron C, Coté R, et al: Extreme temperament and diagnosis: a study in a psychiatric sample of consecutive children. Arch Gen Psychiatry 47:477–484, 1990

McCrae RR, Costa PT: Personality trait structure as a human universal. Am Psychol 52:509–516, 1997

McGuffin P, Thapar A: The genetics of personality disorder. Br J Psychiatry 160:12–23, 1992

Monroe SM, Simons AD: Diathesis-stress theories in the context of life stress research. Psychol Bull 110:406–425, 1991

Nigg JT, Goldsmith HH: Genetics of personality disorders: perspectives from personality and psychopathology research. Psychol Bull 115:346–380, 1994

O'Leary KM, Cowdry RW: Neuropsychological testing results with patients with borderline personality disorder, in Biological and Neurobehavioral Studies of Borderline Personality Disorder. Edited by Silk KR. Washington, DC, American Psychiatric Press, 1994, pp 127–158

Paris J: Borderline Personality Disorder: A Multidimensional Approach. Washington, DC, American Psychiatric Press, 1994

Paris J: Social Factors in the Personality Disorders. New York, Cambridge University Press, 1996

Paris J: Working With Traits. Northvale, NJ, Jason Aronson, 1998

Paris J: Nature and Nurture in Psychiatry. Washington, DC, American Psychiatric Press (in press)

Paykel ES, Cooper Z: Life events, in Handbook of Affective Disorders, 2nd Edition. Edited by Paykel E. New York, Guilford, 1992, pp 149–170

Plomin R, DeFries JC, McClearn GE, et al: Behavioral Genetics: A Primer. New York, WH Freeman, 1997

Reiss D, Plomin R, Hetherington EM: Genetics and psychiatry: an unheralded window on the environment. Am J Psychiatry 149:147–155, 1992

Robins LN: Deviant Children Grown Up. Baltimore, Williams & Wilkins, 1966

Robins LN, Regier DA (eds): Psychiatric Disorders in America. New York, Free Press, 1991

Rutter M: Psychosocial resilience and protective mechanisms. Am J Orthopsychiatry 57:316–331, 1987a

Rutter M: Temperament, personality, and personality development. Br J Psychiatry 150:443–448, 1987b

Rutter M, Quinton D: Long-term follow-up of women institutionalized in childhood. British Journal of Developmental Psychology 18:225–234, 1984

Sato T, Takeichi M: Lifetime prevalence of specific psychiatric disorders in a general medicine clinic. Gen Hosp Psychiatry 15:224–233, 1993

Schneier FR, Spitzer RL, Gibbon M, et al: The relationship of social phobia subtypes and avoidant personality disorder. Compr Psychiatry 32:496–502, 1991

Siever LJ, Davis L: A psychobiological perspective on the personality disorders. Am J Psychiatry 148:1647–1658, 1991

Soloff PH: Psychopharmacological intervention in borderline personality disorder, in Borderline Personality Disorder: Etiology and Treatment. Edited by Paris J. Washington, DC, American Psychiatric Press, 1993, pp 319–348

Soloff PH: Chemotherapy for personality disorder. Paper presented at the 5th International Congress on the Disorders of the Personality. Vancouver, BC, June 25–27, 1997

Soloff PH: Psychopharmacological approaches to the personality disorders. Journal of Practical Psychiatry and Behavioral Health (in press)

Sulloway F: Born to Rebel. New York, Pantheon, 1996

True WR, Rice J, Eisen SA, et al: A twin study of genetic and environmental contributions to liability for post-traumatic stress symptoms. Arch Gen Psychiatry 50:257–264, 1993

Weinberger DR: Implications of normal brain development for the pathogenesis of schizophrenia. Arch Gen Psychiatry 44:660–669

Werner EE, Smith RS: Overcoming the Odds: High Risk Children From Birth to Adulthood. Ithaca, NY, Cornell University Press, 1992

Westen D: Divergences between clinical and research methods for assessing personality disorders: implications for research and the evolution of Axis II. Am J Psychiatry 152:1705–1713, 1997

Yehuda R, McFarlane AC: Conflict between current knowledge about posttraumatic stress disorder and its original conceptual basis. Am J Psychiatry 154:895–903, 1995

Afterword

Kenneth R. Silk, M.D.

The diagnosis of a specific personality disorder often is uncertain, and the treatment is fraught with frustration because of our limited knowledge and even more limited clinical therapeutic applications. Because of these limitations, affected patients have frequently been labeled with negative adjectives such as bad, untreatable, manipulative, sadistic, seductive, and other less-than-complimentary terms. Such terms represent biases among mental health professionals that unfortunately are too widely held, disseminated, and repeated. For this reason, many people avoid considering a personality disorder diagnosis (claiming that the diagnosis is inaccurate or useless) or refuse to treat anyone who would carry such a diagnosis. To the patient who has received such a diagnosis, the label of personality disorder means that someone has seen them as hopeless, difficult, and untreatable.

The way to ameliorate these biases about personality disorders is no different from the way to cure or change any bias in any culture—that is, through education and understanding. The chapters that make up this text and the research and researchers who make up the extensive bibliography listed with each of the chapters might be viewed as the cadre of educators whose role may eventually be to diminish the bias through providing knowledge about personality disorders.

A century of psychological theory with respect to the personality disorders has done much to educate us about how such patients experience the world and their inner lives. As we delve into the biology of neurotransmitters and into polymorphic genes that may greatly influence behavior, we have the beginnings of a new approach to the understanding of these complex disorders and the people who suffer from them. Hopefully, then, continuing biological exploration of the personality disorders will not only provide us with new and valuable information that will inform and direct ever more sophisticated and specific psychiatric treatments but also supply us and others with knowledge that might begin to erode the strong biases and negative labels that have for too long been inappropriately used to describe these troubled, pained human beings.

Index

Page numbers in **boldface** type refer to figures or tables.